Non-Polypoid (Flat and Depressed) Colorectal Neoplasms

Guest Editors

ROY SOETIKNO, MD
TONYA KALTENBACH, MD

GASTROINTESTINAL ENDOSCOPY CLINICS OF NORTH AMERICA

www.giendo.theclinics.com

Consulting Editor
CHARLES J. LIGHTDALE, MD

July 2010 • Volume 20 • Number 3

SAUNDERS an imprint of ELSEVIER, Inc.

W.B. SAUNDERS COMPANY
A Division of Elsevier Inc.

1600 John F. Kennedy Blvd. • Suite 1800 • Philadelphia, Pennsylvania 19103-2899

http://www.giendo.theclinics.com

GASTROINTESTINAL ENDOSCOPY CLINICS OF NORTH AMERICA Volume 20, Number 3
July 2010 ISSN 1052-5157, ISBN-13: 978-1-4377-2526-1

Editor: Kerry Holland
Developmental Editor: Theresa Collier

Gastrointestinal Endoscopy Clinics of North America (ISSN 1052-5157) is published quarterly by Elsevier Inc., 360 Park Avenue South, New York, NY 10010-1710. Months of issue are January, April, July, and October. Business and Editorial Offices: 1600 John F. Kennedy Blvd., Suite 1800, Philadelphia, PA, 19103-2899. Periodicals postage paid at New York, NY and additional mailing offices. Subscription prices are $290.00 per year for US individuals, $394.00 per year for US institutions, $149.00 per year for US students and residents, $320.00 per year for Canadian individuals, $481.00 per year for Canadian institutions, $405.00 per year for international individuals, $481.00 per year for international institutions, and $207.00 per year for Canadian and foreign students/residents. To receive student/resident rate, orders must be accompanied by name of affiliated institution, date of term, and the signature of program/residency coordinator on institution letterhead. Orders will be billed at individual rate until proof of status is received. Foreign air speed delivery is included in all Clinics subscription prices. All prices are subject to change without notice. POSTMASTER: Send address change to Gastrointestinal Endoscopy Clinics of North America, Elsevier Health Sciences Division, Subscription Customer Service, 3251 Riverport Lane, Maryland Heights, MO 63043. Customer Service: 1-800-654-2452 (US). From outside the United States, call 1-314-447-8871. Fax: 1-314-447-8029. E-mail: JournalsCustomerService-usa@elsevier.com (for print support) or JournalsOnlineSupport-usa@elsevier.com (for online support).

Reprints. For copies of 100 or more, of articles in this publication, please contact the Commercial Reprints Department, Elsevier Inc., 360 Park Avenue South, New York, NY 10010-1710. Tel. (212) 633-3812; Fax: (212) 482-1935; E-mail: reprints@elsevier.com.

Gastrointestinal Endoscopy Clinics of North America is covered in Excerpta Medica, MEDLINE/PubMed (Index Medicus), and MEDLINE/MEDLARS.

Printed and bound by CPI Group (UK) Ltd, Croydon, CR0 4YY
Transferred to Digital Print 2011

Contributors

CONSULTING EDITOR

CHARLES J. LIGHTDALE, MD
Professor, Department of Medicine, Columbia University Medical Center, New York, New York

GUEST EDITORS

ROY SOETIKNO, MD
Chief of Endoscopy, Veterans Affairs Palo Alto Health Care System; and Clinical Professor of Medicine (Affiliated), Stanford University School of Medicine, Palo Alto, California

TONYA KALTENBACH, MD
Clinician, Veterans Affairs Palo Alto Health Care System; and Clinical Assistant Professor of Medicine (Affiliated), Stanford University School of Medicine, Palo Alto, California

AUTHORS

DAVID BURLING, MD, MRCP, FRCP
Department of Intestinal Imaging, St Marks Hospital, Harrow, Middlesex, United Kingdom

KAZUAKI CHAYAMA, MD, PhD
Professor, Department of Medicine and Molecular Science, Hiroshima University, Hiroshima, Japan

TAKAHIRO FUJII, MD, PhD
Fujii Takahiro Clinic, Chuo-ku, Tokyo, Japan

JOHN HART, MD
Professor of Pathology, Department of Pathology, University of Chicago Medical Center, Chicago, Illinois

DAVID G. HEWETT, MBBS, FRACP
Division of Gastroenterology and Hepatology, Department of Medicine, Indiana University School of Medicine, Indianapolis, Indiana

ANA IGNJATOVIC, BA, BMBCh, MRCP
Research Fellow, Wolfson Unit for Endoscopy, Imperial College, St Mark's Hospital, London, United Kingdom

MINEO IWADATE, MD
Gastrointestinal Center, Sano Hospital, Tarumi-ku, Kobe, Hyogo, Japan

CHARLES J. KAHI, MD, MSc, FACP
Associate Professor of Clinical Medicine, Division of Gastroenterology and Hepatology, Department of Medicine, Indiana University School of Medicine; Gastroenterology Section Chief, Roudebush, Veterans Affairs Medical Center, Indianapolis, Indiana

LYN SUE KAHNG, MD
Assistant Professor of Medicine, Section of Digestive Diseases and Nutrition, University of Illinois at Chicago and Jesse Brown Veterans Affairs Medical Center, Chicago, Illinois

TONYA KALTENBACH, MD
Clinician, Veterans Affairs Palo Alto Health Care System; and Clinical Assistant Professor of Medicine (Affiliated), Stanford University School of Medicine, Palo Alto, California

H.N. KIM, MD
Department of Gastroenterology, Hepatology, and Nutrition, The University of Texas M.D. Anderson Cancer Center, Houston, Texas

NOZOMU KOBAYASHI, MD
Department of Diagnostic Imaging, Tochigi Cancer Center, Tochigi, Japan

AD A.M. MASCLEE, MD, PhD
Department of Internal Medicine, Division of Gastroenterology and Hepatology, Maastricht University Medical Center, Maastricht, The Netherlands

TAKAHISA MATSUDA, MD, PhD
Endoscopy Division, National Cancer Center Hospital, Chuo-ku, Tokyo, Japan

TAKESHI NAKAJIMA, MD, PhD
Endoscopy Division, National Cancer Center Hospital, Chuo-ku, Tokyo, Japan

AMY E. NOFFSINGER, MD
Professor of Pathology, Department of Pathology, University of Cincinnati, Cincinnati, Ohio

ADOLFO PARRA-BLANCO, MD, PhD
Department of Gastroenterology, Central University Hospital of Asturias, Oviedo, Spain

G.S. RAJU, MD, FASGE
Department of Gastroenterology, Hepatology, and Nutrition, The University of Texas M.D. Anderson Cancer Center, Houston, Texas

DOUGLAS K. REX, MD
Distinguished Professor of Medicine, Division of Gastroenterology and Hepatology, Department of Medicine, Indiana University School of Medicine, Indianapolis, Indiana

EVELINE J.A. RONDAGH, MD
Department of Internal Medicine, Division of Gastroenterology and Hepatology, Maastricht University Medical Center, Maastricht, The Netherlands

YUTAKA SAITO, MD, PhD
Endoscopy Division, National Cancer Center Hospital, Chuo-ku, Tokyo, Japan

TAKU SAKAMOTO, MD
Endoscopy Division, National Cancer Center Hospital, Chuo-ku, Tokyo, Japan

SILVIA SANDULEANU, MD, PhD
Department of Internal Medicine, Division of Gastroenterology and Hepatology, Maastricht University Medical Center, Maastricht, The Netherlands

YASUSHI SANO, MD, PhD
Director and Chief, Gastrointestinal Center, Sano Hospital, Tarumi-ku, Kobe, Hyogo, Japan

BRIAN P. SAUNDERS, MD, FRCP
Reader in Endoscopy, Imperial College; Director, Wolfson Unit for Endoscopy, Imperial College, St Mark's Hospital, London, United Kingdom

ROY SOETIKNO, MD
Chief of Endoscopy, Veterans Affairs Palo Alto Health Care System; and Clinical Professor of Medicine (Affiliated), Stanford University School of Medicine, Palo Alto, California

NORIKO SUZUKI, MD, PhD
Wolfson Unit for Endoscopy, St Mark's Hospital, Harrow, Middlesex, United Kingdom

SHINJI TANAKA, MD, PhD
Professor, Department of Endoscopy, Hiroshima University Hospital, Hiroshima, Japan

STUART A. TAYLOR, MD, MRCP, FRCP
Department of Specialist Imaging, University College Hospital, London, United Kingdom

YOSHITAKA UENO, MD, PhD
Physician, Department of Endoscopy, Hiroshima University Hospital, Hiroshima, Japan

THOMAS D. WANG, MD, PhD
Assistant Professor, Division of Gastroenterology and Hepatology, Department of Medicine, University of Michigan School of Medicine; Assistant Professor, Department of Biomedical Engineering, University of Michigan, Ann Arbor, Michigan

Contents

Foreword   xiii

Charles J. Lightdale

Preface   xv

Roy Soetikno and Tonya Kaltenbach

Relationship of Non-Polypoid Colorectal Neoplasms to Quality of Colonoscopy   407

Charles J. Kahi, David G. Hewett, and Douglas K. Rex

> Colonoscopy is a dominant modality for colorectal cancer prevention in average-risk patients aged 50 years and older. Non-polypoid colorectal neoplasms (NP-CRNs) are likely a significant contributing factor to interval colorectal cancers because they have a higher prevalence in Western populations than previously thought, are more difficult to detect visually with conventional colonoscopy, and are more likely to contain advanced histology than polypoid neoplasms, regardless of size. The accurate identification and complete removal of NP-CRNs is thus an integral part of high-quality colonoscopy, and a critical component of the ongoing efforts to make colorectal cancer screening programs widely available, effective, and accepted by patients. In this article, the authors examine the quality indicators for colonoscopy, present the reasons for interval cancers, and discuss the relation between NP-CRNs and quality colonoscopy.

Non-Polypoid Colorectal Neoplasms are Relatively Common Worldwide   417

Ana Ignjatovic and Brian P. Saunders

> Flat adenomas are found commonly at colonoscopy throughout the world. Similarly, small, flat submucosally invasive cancers have been described worldwide but are relatively rare, accounting for 5% to 10% of all cancers detected at colonoscopy. Although there appears to be no difference in frequency of non-polypoid colorectal neoplasms between East and West, considerable variation has been reported by individual studies, probably because of lack of consistency when defining a flat lesion. Flat elevated lesions are the most common type of flat lesion and do not appear to have a greatly increased risk of harboring invasive malignancy; however, flat lesions with depression have a significant risk of malignancy and are probably the precursor lesions for most small, flat, or ulcerating cancers.

The Natural History of Non-Polypoid Colorectal Neoplasms   431

Nozomu Kobayashi, Takahisa Matsuda, and Yasushi Sano

> Despite their importance, little is known about the natural history of non-polypoid colorectal neoplasms (NP-CRN). This article will summarize the available data to gain some estimates of the natural history of NP-CRN.

Bowel Preparation and Colonoscopy Technique To Detect Non-Polypoid Colorectal Neoplasms   437

H.N. Kim and G.S. Raju

Colonoscopy is considered the gold standard for colon cancer screening. In a recent study, however, 0.3% to 0.9% patients developed colorectal cancer within 3 years after removal of adenomas. Some reasons for the development of interval colorectal cancers include missed or incompletely removed lesions during the initial colonoscopy. Non-polypoid colorectal neoplasms are a potential contributor to the pool of missed lesions because they can be easily missed as a result of inadequate colon preparation or examination technique. This article discusses the methods that are useful to improve the quality of bowel preparation and examination technique.

Development of Expertise in the Detection and Classification of Non-Polypoid Colorectal Neoplasia: Experience-Based Data at an Academic GI Unit   449

Silvia Sanduleanu, Eveline J.A. Rondagh, and Ad A.M. Masclee

At its core, quality improvement in gastrointestinal (GI) practice relies on continuous training, education, and information among all health care providers, whether gastroenterologists, GI trainees, endoscopy nurses, or GI pathologists. Over the past few years, it became clear that objective criteria are needed to assess the quality of colonoscopy, such as cecum intubation rate, quality of bowel preparation, withdrawal time, and adenoma detection rate. In this context, development of competence among practicing endoscopists to adequately detect and treat non-polypoid colorectal neoplasms (NP-CRNs) deserves special attention. We describe a summary of the path to develop expertise in detection and management of NP-CRNs, based on experience at our academic GI unit.

The Importance of the Macroscopic Classification of Colorectal Neoplasms   461

Yasushi Sano and Mineo Iwadate

The importance and prevalence of the superficial lesions in the colon and rectum caught worldwide public attention in 2008 when Soetikno and colleagues reported the prevalence of non-polypoid (flat and depressed) colorectal neoplasms in asymptomatic and symptomatic adults in North America and the public media disseminated their findings. The publication put to rest the question of whether or not the flat and depressed colorectal neoplasms exist in Western countries; flat and depressed colorectal neoplasms can be found throughout the world. In this article, the author highlights the importance of the macroscopic classification of the colorectal neoplasm and emphasizes the distinction between so-called flat lesions (IIa and IIb) and 0-IIc (superficial depressed) neoplastic colorectal lesions.

Image-Enhanced Endoscopy Is Critical in the Detection, Diagnosis, and Treatment of Non-Polypoid Colorectal Neoplasms   471

Tonya Kaltenbach and Roy Soetikno

Colonoscopy, the most sensitive test used to detect advanced adenoma and cancer, has been shown to prevent colorectal cancer (CRC) when combined with polypectomy. CRC remains the third most commonly diagnosed cancer and the second leading cause of cancer death in men and women in the United States. Image-enhanced endoscopy (IEE) is an integral part in the detection, diagnosis, and treatment of non-polypoid colorectal neoplasms. Both the dye-based and equipment-based varieties of IEE are readily available for application in today's practice of colonoscopy. Data are available to support its use, although further studies are needed to simplify the classification of colorectal lesions by the different techniques of equipment-based IEE.

Assessment of Likelihood of Submucosal Invasion in Non-Polypoid Colorectal Neoplasms   487

Takahisa Matsuda, Adolfo Parra-Blanco, Yutaka Saito, Taku Sakamoto, and Takeshi Nakajima

Although of lower prevalence compared with polypoid neoplasms, the non-polypoid neoplasms, especially the depressed type, are important to diagnose because they belong to a distinct biologically aggressive subset, given the high rate of intramucosal or submucosal cancers. The detection and diagnosis of the non-polypoid colorectal neoplasm presents a challenge and an opportunity. Above all, characteristic colonoscopic findings obtained by a combination of conventional colonoscopy and magnifying chromoendoscopy are useful for determination of the invasion depth of non-polypoid colorectal cancers, an essential factor in selecting a treatment modality.

Dynamic Submucosal Injection Technique   497

Roy Soetikno and Tonya Kaltenbach

This article describes the submucosal injection technique applied in the endoscopic resection of non-polypoid colorectal neoplasms, with an emphasis on a particular technique, the dynamic submucosal injection technique.

Endoscopic Mucosal Resection of Non-Polypoid Colorectal Neoplasm   503

Tonya Kaltenbach and Roy Soetikno

Endoscopic mucosal resection (EMR) is preferred to standard polypectomy for the resection of non-polypoid lesions because these lesions can be technically difficult to capture with a snare; furthermore, without submucosal injection the underlying muscularis propria may be excessively coagulated or even inadvertently resected. Because the resection plane of EMR is in the middle or deeper part of the submucosa, EMR allows the precise depth of the lesion to be evaluated. Although the majority of non-polypoid lesions are adenomatous, non-polypoid colorectal neoplasm has a high association with advanced pathology, irrespective of size. Using EMR, a complete pathologic specimen is obtained, the risk of lymph node metastasis can be accurately assessed based on the depth of invasion, and patients can be suitably managed. Used according to its indications, EMR provides curative resection, and obviates the higher morbidity, mortality, and cost associated with surgical treatment.

Endoscopic Submucosal Dissection of Non-Polypoid Colorectal Neoplasms   515

Yutaka Saito, Takahisa Matsuda, and Takahiro Fujii

> Traditionally, endoscopic mucosal resection and surgery were the only available treatments for large colorectal tumors, even for those detected at an early stage. The endoscopic submucosal dissection (ESD) technique, which enables en-bloc resection of large tumors, is accepted as a standard minimally invasive treatment for early gastric cancer in Japan. This article explains in detail how ESD is performed and compares it with endoscopic mucosal resection.

Non-Polypoid Colorectal Neoplasms in Ulcerative Colitis   525

Yoshitaka Ueno, Shinji Tanaka, and Kazuaki Chayama

> The incidence of colorectal cancer associated with ulcerative colitis (UC) increases with time. It is imperative to identify dysplasia-associated lesions or masses (DALM) and non-polypoid colorectal neoplasms (NP-CRN) to reduce the morbidity and mortality from colorectal cancer associated with UC. Recent findings suggest most dysplastic lesions in UC can be considered as visible under careful endoscopic observation. To find NP-CRN in UC, the careful examination of well-prepared mucosa and noting subtle differences is necessary. Magnifying chromoendoscopy, therefore, can be useful to endoscopically diagnose these subtle findings. The authors believe that targeted biopsies during chromoendoscopy will increasingly be used and replace random biopsies in the future.

Serrated Adenoma: A Distinct Form of Non-Polypoid Colorectal Neoplasia?   543

Amy E. Noffsinger and John Hart

> Until recently, 2 major forms of colorectal polyp were recognized: the adenoma and the hyperplastic polyp. Adenomas were known to represent a precursor to colorectal cancer, whereas hyperplastic polyps were viewed as nonneoplastic, having no potential for progression to malignancy. We now recognize, however, that the lesions diagnosed as hyperplastic polyps in the past represent a heterogeneous group of polyps, some of which truly are hyperplastic, and others that truly have a significant risk for transformation to colorectal cancer. These polyps have a characteristic serrated architecture, and include not only hyperplastic polyps but also the recently recognized serrated adenomas. Serrated adenomas occur in 2 forms: the traditional serrated adenoma, which is usually a polypoid lesion endoscopically, and the sessile serrated adenoma, a flat or slightly raised, usually right-sided lesion. Serrated adenomas of both types show characteristic molecular alterations not commonly seen in traditional colorectal adenomas, and probably progress to colorectal cancer by means of a different pathway, the so-called serrated neoplasia pathway. The morphologic features of serrated colorectal lesions, the molecular alterations that characterize them, and their role in colorectal cancer development are discussed.

CT Colonography and Non-Polypoid Colorectal Neoplasms   565

Noriko Suzuki, Ana Ignjatovic, David Burling, and Stuart A. Taylor

> Computed tomographic colonography (CTC) has been reported to be as effective as optical colonoscopy in the detection of significant adenomas.

However, there are widely conflicting performance data in relation to detection of flat neoplasia. This article describes the potential and limitations of CTC and computer-aided diagnosis in the detection of flat neoplasms.

Genetic Aspects of Non-Polypoid Colorectal Neoplasms   573

Lyn Sue Kahng

Colorectal cancer is a heterogeneous disease arising through multiple possible pathways. Elucidating the genetic factors controlling molecular phenotype, morphology, histology, and prognosis of different tumor types continues to be a challenge. Non-polypoid colorectal neoplasms provide opportunities for ongoing study of their underlying genetic abnormalities and molecular phenotypes. The varied data from different groups, however, highlight the need for further studies in different populations.

Targeted Imaging of Flat and Depressed Colonic Neoplasms   579

Thomas D. Wang

Molecular imaging is a rapidly growing new discipline in gastrointestinal endoscopy that involves the development of novel imaging probes and instruments to visualize the molecular expression pattern of mucosa in the digestive tract. Several platforms for imaging agents, including antibody and peptide, are being developed to target over expressed biomolecules in cancer. In addition, novel imaging instruments, including fluorescence endoscopy and confocal microscopy, are being developed to provide wide-area surveillance and microscopic examination, respectively. These methods are being applied to detect the presence of flat and depressed colonic neoplasms and to identify tumor margins.

Index   585

FORTHCOMING ISSUES

October 2010
Quality Colonoscopy
John I. Allen, MD, *Guest Editor*

January 2011
Advances in the Diagnosis and Management
of Barrett's Esophagus
Irving Waxman, MD, *Guest Editor*

April 2011
Bariatrics for the Endoscopist
Christopher C. Thompson, MD,
Guest Editor

RECENT ISSUES

April 2010
CT Colonography
Subhas Banerjee, MD and
Jacques Van Dam, MD, PhD, *Guest Editors*

January 2010
Endoluminal Therapy for Esophageal Disease
Herbert C. Wolfsen, MD, *Guest Editor*

October 2009
Intraductal Biliary and Pancreatic Endoscopy
Peter D. Stevens, MD, *Guest Editor*

THE CLINICS ARE NOW AVAILABLE ONLINE!
Access your subscription at:
www.theclinics.com

Foreword

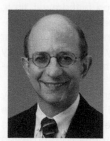

Charles J. Lightdale, MD
   Consulting Editor

Every once in a while the publication of a single clinical research article can have a tremendously powerful effect by shining a bright light on a shadowed area. The article can provoke widespread discussion and reassessment of clinical practice, and can be a key factor in galvanizing changes leading to improved outcomes. Such an article was published in the *Journal of the American Medical Association* on March 5, 2008, and the lead author was Dr Roy M. Soetikno, the Guest Editor for this issue of the *Gastrointestinal Endoscopy Clinics of North America* dedicated to "non-polypoid colorectal neoplasms."[1] It demonstrated in 1819 patients evaluated in the Veterans Affairs Palo Alto (California) Health Care System, in the year July 2003 to June 2004, that non-polypoid neoplasms in the colon were not rare in the United States. On the contrary, the study showed that what many specialists in the United States were dismissing as a "Japanese disease" was quite common among American veterans: 9.35% overall, and 15.44% in the group undergoing surveillance colonoscopy.

Dr Soetikno and colleagues not only found that non-polypoid lesions were relatively common, but that they were five times more likely to contain carcinoma than polypoid lesions irrespective of size. The depressed-type adenoma was the least common, but had the highest risk of containing cancer (33%), confirming what Japanese investigators had observed for decades. My own exposure to this concept was from several encounters with Professor Shin-ei Kudo in the 1990s, including an intensive educational program in Yokohama. I wrote a book review for *Gastrointestinal Endoscopy* in 1998[2] praising his English language book *Early colorectal cancer: detection of depressed types of colorectal carcinoma*.[3] The Kudo classification of mucosal pit patterns of colon lesions remains a widely used standard.

The article by Soetikno and colleagues[1] shattered the last resistance to the acceptance of the importance of non-polypoid lesions in the colon. Although colon cancer prevention and early detection with colonoscopy screening in the United States has resulted in enormous benefit, studies have shown that from 0.3% to 0.9% of patients develop colon cancers within a few years of having a colonoscopy. It seems highly probable that flat lesions missed or incompletely removed at colonoscopy may account for some of these failures.

doi:10.1016/j.giec.2010.05.002

The finding of the relatively common prevalence of non-polypoid lesions in the United States also joined with other studies relating to the accuracy of colonoscopy, including the importance of preparation quality and endoscope withdrawal time, sparking new approaches to colonoscopy training and practice. Although colonoscopy quality should be improved with training and quality assurance approaches, it is also likely that subtle, flat lesions difficult to see on colonoscopy will almost certainly be missed on CT colonography. Thus, there is another reason to favor optical colonoscopy for screening most populations.

It has become evident to most colonoscopists that pit pattern analysis can be highly accurate, allowing real-time decisions for management. The old adage to "just take a biopsy, and we'll find out later" is being replaced. New high-definition endoscopes with narrow-band imaging or digital chromoendoscopy are making detection and lesion characterization by pit pattern analysis even easier, and new optical methods, such as confocal laser endomicroscopy, may add additional accuracy. Colonoscopists not only have to detect and characterize non-polypoid lesions, but must carefully assess the full extent of lesions, and decide how best to completely remove them. Techniques for en bloc removal of high-risk lesions using endoscopic mucosal resection and endoscopic submucosal dissection are increasingly taught and used. Dr Soetikno has been in the forefront of detection, differentiation, and management of non-polypoid lesions in the colon, and has assembled an extraordinary array of topics and authors, providing a comprehensive review in this landmark issue of the *Gastrointestinal Endoscopy Clinics of North America*. For those performing colonoscopy (and that includes most practicing gastroenterologists), this is a must read.

Charles J. Lightdale, MD
Department of Medicine
Columbia University Medical Center
161 Fort Washington Avenue
Room 812, New York, NY 10032, USA

E-mail address:
CJL18@columbia.edu

REFERENCES

1. Soetikno RM, Kaltenbach T, Rouse RV, et al. Prevalence of non-polypoid (flat and depressed) colorectal neoplasms in asymptomatic and symptomatic adults. JAMA 2008;299:1027–35.
2. Lightdale CJ. Early colorectal cancer: detection of depressed types of colorectal carcinoma [book review]. Gastrointest Endosc 1998;48:338–9.
3. Kudo S. Early colorectal cancer: detection of depressed types of colorectal carcinoma. Igaku-Shoin (Tokyo) and New York, 1996.

Preface

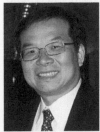 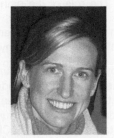

Roy Soetikno, MD   Tonya Kaltenbach, MD
Guest Editors

"Here's to the crazy ones. The misfits. The rebels. The troublemakers. The round pegs in the square holes. The ones who see things differently. They're not fond of rules. And they have no respect for the status quo. You can quote them, disagree with them, glorify or vilify them. About the only thing you can't do is ignore them. Because they change things. They push the human race forward. And while some may see them as the crazy ones, we see genius. Because the people who are crazy enough to think they can change the world, are the ones who do."
Authored by Steve Jobs - according to Apple folklore..

The recognition of the importance of the non-polypoid colorectal neoplasms (NP-CRNs) is an important step in the efforts to improving the quality of endoscopy for the prevention of colorectal cancer. Without this step many pre- or early cancerous lesions may not be sought after and removed. Furthermore, the detection, diagnosis, and resections techniques of pre- and early cancer, which provides the best chance of survival, will not be learned and taught for the benefit of more patients. We thank Dr David Lieberman for his insights for quoting Sir James Dewar, "People's minds are like parachutes—they only function when they open," in his eloquent editorial about the importance and significance of NP-CRNs. The need to have an open mind cannot be emphasized further as we are still in the beginning phase of understanding NP-CRNs and incorporating it into practice.

We are pleased to have continuing interest and support from reporters and editors from local, national, and international media, who disseminated the findings of the existence and significance of NP-CRNs at the Veterans Affairs Palo Alto to the general public. Their efforts have helped to open many more minds about the importance of quality colonoscopy and the contribution of subtle lesions, such as NP-CRNs, to the development of colorectal cancer. The widespread detection and management of NP-CRNs, however, requires the medical field to implement several paradigm shift concepts:

1. Detection of pre- and early colorectal neoplasms: to search for an abnormal patch of mucosa with and without image-enhanced endoscopy rather than to focus only on detecting a protruding lesion.

Gastrointest Endoscopy Clin N Am 20 (2010) xv–xvi
doi:10.1016/j.giec.2010.05.001
1052-5157/10/$ – see front matter

2. Diagnosis of pre- and early colorectal neoplasms: to use the endoscope to diagnose lesions at the time of endoscopy to make treatment decisions rather than to rely on the pathology of a specimen. The role of the pathology is to confirm the endoscopic diagnosis.
3. Treatment of pre- and early colorectal neoplasms: to use endoscopic mucosal resection techniques routinely rather than simple polypectomy alone.

In this issue of *Gastrointestinal Endoscopy Clinics of North America*, we, with the contributors, wish to describe these concepts in detail. We provide a practical collection of information for endoscopists to detect, diagnose, and treat more NP-CRNs in their practice. We thank Dr Charles Lightdale for the opportunity to publish this descriptive collection of the current understanding of the NP-CRNs. We thank the contributing authors immensely. We wish to acknowledge the assistance of Kerry Holland of Elsevier, who made it possible for this issue to have many colorful images.

Although the preparation of this issue took a mere few months, its groundwork took more than a decade and required the input of many. Through innumerable visits to units in Japan, Europe, and the United States itself, we have learned from their mastery of endoscopy—it is impossible to mention them one by one. We do thank, in particular, the many endoscopists and pathologists of the endoscopy division of the National Cancer Center hospital in Tsukiji, Japan, formerly led by Drs Takahiro Fujii and Tadakazu Shimoda, for their tireless efforts to disseminate knowledge of NP-CRNs worldwide. We thank our colleagues from the Interdisciplinary Endoscopy Department and Clinic, Universitätsklinikum Hamburg-Eppendorf, formerly led by Dr Nib Soehendra, for sharing useful resection techniques and the use of endoscopic clipping to treat its potential complications. The fundamental principle—that has been a continuing source of inspiration and ultimately led to our study of NP-CRNs—was taught by Dr Michael Blackstone, formerly of the University of Chicago. He instilled the importance of interpreting what we see during endoscopy (rather than waiting for pathology results). Lastly, we appreciate our patients for allowing us to learn from them and our supportive staff and colleagues, led by Elizabeth Freeman, and Drs Lawrence Leung and Stephen Ezeji-Okoye—without them we would not have been able to put together this issue.

Roy Soetikno, MD
Veterans Affairs Palo Alto Health Care System
3801 Miranda Avenue, GI-111
Palo Alto, CA 94304, USA

Tonya Kaltenbach, MD
Veterans Affairs Palo Alto Health Care System
3801 Miranda Avenue, GI-111
Palo Alto, CA 94304, USA

E-mail addresses:
soetikno@earthlink.net (R. Soetikno)
tonya_kolodziejski@yahoo.com (T. Kaltenbach)

Relationship of Non-Polypoid Colorectal Neoplasms to Quality of Colonoscopy

Charles J. Kahi, MD, MSc*, David G. Hewett, MBBS, FRACP, Douglas K. Rex, MD

KEYWORDS

- Non-polypoid colorectal neoplasms • Colonoscopy
- Colorectal cancer • Adenoma

Colonoscopy is a dominant modality for colorectal cancer (CRC) prevention in average-risk patients aged 50 years and older. The principal benefits of screening colonoscopy are that it allows complete examination of the colon, detection of colorectal neoplasms, removal of polyps, and risk stratification of patients according to colorectal neoplasia type and burden.[1] Screening colonoscopy identifies patients with no adenomas who can then be selected for longer surveillance intervals; patients with adenomas who can undergo polypectomy, and the small subgroup of patients with clinically silent early stage CRC. Despite its positive impact on CRC incidence and mortality, colonoscopy affords imperfect protection because some patients are diagnosed with CRC after a short time interval (1 to 3 years) following colonoscopy with potentially devastating impact on patients and colonoscopists.[2] There are several potential explanations for the failure of clearing colonoscopy to prevent interval cancers, including patient factors, such as inadequate bowel preparation and variation in tumor biology; and physician factors, such as suboptimal withdrawal, examination, polypectomy techniques, and perceptual and personality attributes. Non-polypoid colorectal neoplasms (NP-CRNs) are likely a significant contributing factor to interval CRCs because they have a higher prevalence in Western populations than previously thought, are more difficult to detect visually with conventional colonoscopy, and are more likely to contain advanced histology than polypoid

Division of Gastroenterology and Hepatology, Department of Medicine, Indiana University School of Medicine, Indianapolis, IN, USA
* Corresponding author. Roudebush Veterans Affairs Medical Center, 1481 West 10th Street, 111G, Indianapolis, IN 46202.
E-mail address: ckahi2@iupui.edu

Gastrointest Endoscopy Clin N Am 20 (2010) 407–415
doi:10.1016/j.giec.2010.03.001
1052-5157/10/$ – see front matter. Published by Elsevier Inc.

giendo.theclinics.com

neoplasms, regardless of size.[3] The accurate identification and complete removal of NP-CRNs is thus an integral part of high-quality colonoscopy, and a critical component of the ongoing efforts to make CRC screening programs widely available, effective, and accepted by patients. In this article, the authors examine the quality indicators for colonoscopy, present the reasons for interval cancers, and discuss the relation between NP-CRNs and quality colonoscopy.

QUALITY INDICATORS FOR COLONOSCOPY

The quality indicators for colonoscopy can be broadly categorized into pre-procedure, intra-procedure, and post-procedure indicators (**Box 1**).[4] The indicators most relevant to NP-CRNs are bowel preparation quality, detection of adenomas in asymptomatic individuals, withdrawal time, and complete endoscopic resection of polyps. Suboptimal bowel preparation hinders the adequate performance of colonoscopy because it can prolong procedure time (during insertion and withdrawal), and is associated with a lower detection rate of small[5] and large adenomas.[5,6] At least one prospective study found that improved bowel preparation preferentially increased the detection of flat lesions,[7] a result that seems intuitively logical because NP-CRNs are more difficult to detect given their small size and flat morphology. The impact of prolonged procedure time on colonoscopy quality and operator fatigue is difficult to quantify. However, studies have shown that cecal intubation rates decline and insertion times tend to

---

Box 1
Quality indicators for colonoscopy

1. Appropriate indication

2. Informed consent is obtained, including specific discussion of risks associated with colonoscopy

3. Use of recommended post-polypectomy and post-cancer resection surveillance intervals

4. Use of recommended ulcerative colitis/Crohn's disease surveillance intervals

5. Documentation in the procedure note of the quality of the preparation

6. Cecal intubation rates (visualization of the cecum by notation of landmarks and photo documentation of landmarks should be present in every procedure)

7. Detection of adenomas in asymptomatic individuals (screening)

8. Withdrawal time: mean withdrawal time should be greater than or equal to 6 minutes in colonoscopies with normal results performed in patients with intact anatomy

9. Biopsy specimens obtained in patients with chronic diarrhea

10. Number and distribution of biopsy samples in ulcerative colitis and Crohn's colitis surveillance (goal: four per 10-cm section of involved colon or approximately 32 specimens per case of pancolitis)

11. Mucosally based pedunculated polyps and sessile polyps less than 2 cm in size should be endoscopically resected or if unresectable, documentation should be obtained

12. Incidence of perforation by procedure type (all indications vs screening) is measured

13. Incidence of post-polypectomy bleeding is measured

14. Nonoperative management of Post-polypectomy bleeding

Data from Rex DK, Petrini JL, Baron TH, et al. Quality indicators for colonoscopy. Gastrointest Endosc 2006;63:S16.

lengthen with consecutive colonoscopies,[8] and adenoma detection rates are higher for colonoscopies performed in the morning compared with ones performed later in the day.[9] Thus, an inadequate bowel preparation, beyond the obvious deleterious effect on visualization, may have an adverse impact on the vigilance of colonoscopists because of fatigue or other factors leading to decreased adenoma detection rates for procedures performed later in the day.

The measurement of adenoma detection rates of individual endoscopists is a central component of the colonoscopy quality monitoring process, given that the detection and removal of precancerous adenomas is one of the fundamental goals of colonoscopy.[4] The minimum adenoma detection rates in healthy, asymptomatic patients aged 50 years or older who are undergoing screening colonoscopy are 25% for men and 15% for women. Similar detection thresholds specific for NP-CRNs have not been defined, largely because this requires knowledge of the true prevalence of these neoplasms in average-risk populations. The relation between the prevalence of NP-CRNs in Western populations and overall adenoma detection rates is discussed later.

Withdrawal time is a surrogate measure for adequate withdrawal and inspection technique. Withdrawal times of 6 minutes or more are associated with increased detection of adenomas.[10] The effect of withdrawal time on NP-CRN detection is not known.

INTERVAL COLORECTAL CANCERS

Despite the evidence supporting a protective effect of colonoscopy and polypectomy on CRC incidence and mortality, there is increasing evidence that the degree of protection depends on the effectiveness of identification and removal of precursor adenomas. The National Polyp Study (NPS) reported a 76% to 90% reduction in the incidence of CRC in patients with adenomas who underwent colonoscopy and polypectomy, compared with three reference cohorts,[11] with a long-term impact on CRC incidence and mortality, which can be attributed mostly to the baseline colonoscopy.[12] An Italian prospective cohort study, conducted in standard clinical practice, reported findings similar to those of the NPS.[13] Taken together, these studies form the basis of the widely quoted statement that about 80% of CRCs can be prevented by colonoscopy with polypectomy. However, recent adenoma cohort studies have reported lower levels of protection after colonoscopy, especially in the proximal colon. Two dietary fiber trials reported rates of incident CRC after clearing colonoscopy three to four times higher than those in the NPS.[14,15] A study combining the results of three adenoma chemoprevention trials did not report a significant effect on CRC incidence compared with a surveillance, epidemiology and end results reference cohort (standardized incidence ratio 0.98, 95% CI 0.63–1.54).[16] A German population-based case-control study found that subjects with a previous negative colonoscopy had a 74% lower risk for CRC than those without previous colonoscopy, with the risk reduction most marked for subjects with rectal or sigmoid CRCs.[17] A large claims-based Canadian study assessing the incidence of CRC after a negative colonoscopy reported standardized incidence ratios of 0.66 at 1 year, 0.55 at 5 years, and 0.28 at 10 years.[18] The declining incidence ratios over time support the notion that some CRCs were diagnosed soon after the baseline colonoscopy and likely represent latent lesions that were missed during the initial examination. In that study, 47% of the incident CRCs were located in the proximal colon compared with 28% in the distal colon ($P<.001$).[18]

In a case-control study involving 4458 CRCs and 43,815 controls in the California Medicaid population, Singh and colleagues[19] reported that adjusted relative risk for proximal CRC following negative colonoscopy was significantly higher (0.67) than distal CRC (0.16). A widely quoted claims-based case-control study from Canada reported that complete colonoscopy was associated with fewer deaths from left-sided CRC (adjusted conditional odds ratio [OR], 0.33 [CI, 0.28 to 0.39]) but not from right-sided CRC (adjusted conditional OR, 0.99 [CI, 0.86 to 1.14]).[20]

The possible reasons for the occurrence of interval cancers are listed in **Box 2**. Biologic variation in tumor growth likely contributes to interval cancers, especially in the proximal colon and for depressed NP-CRNs; studies have shown that interval cancers, compared with non-interval cancers, are more likely to arise in the proximal colon, demonstrate the CpG island methylator phenotype, and have microsatellite instability.[21,22] However, variable sensitivity caused by operator-dependent inspection quality is also a central factor associated with adenoma detection. The causes listed in **Box 2** are interrelated and it is often challenging to tease out a definite cause for why a specific interval cancer occurred. For example, in a study of 37 interval CRCs (76% proximal), four were in subjects who had failed to present for follow-up, two were likely caused by incomplete polypectomy, and seven had poor bowel preparation at the baseline colonoscopy.[23] In another study, of 830 CRCs diagnosed during the study period, 45 subjects developed an interval cancer (5.4%; 95% CI, 4.1%–7.2%), of which 27% developed at previous polypectomy segments. Interval cancers were three times more likely to occur in the right colon and were smaller in size than sporadic cancers. Quality of bowel preparation, individual endoscopist, endoscopist experience, and trainee involvement were not associated with interval cancers.[24] Other studies have found that proximal CRC, advanced age, diverticular

---

Box 2
Possible reasons for why colonoscopy protection is imperfect

Patient
- Poor bowel preparation
- Tumor biology (including genetic factors and environmental factors, such as diet/ smoking)

Colonoscopist
- Procedural/motor skill deficits (eg, incomplete colonoscopy, incomplete/inadequate polypectomy, withdrawal technique)
- Perceptual factors (eg, variation in color and depth perception)
- Personality characteristics (conscientiousness, obsessiveness, impulsivity)
- Knowledge and attitude deficits (eg, awareness and appearance of flat lesions)

System
- Financial factors (eg, reimbursement disincentives)
- Organizational factors (eg, workload pressures, level of training)

Technical
- Inadequate equipment (eg, poor image resolution)

Data from Hewett DG, Kahi CJ, Rex DK. Does colonoscopy work? The Journal of the National Comprehensive Cancer Network 2010;8(1):67–77; with permission.

disease, colonoscopy by an internist of family physician, and office-based procedure were independent predictors of missed CRC.[25] An analysis of interval cancers in the Polyp Prevention Trial found that more than 50% of 13 interval CRCs could have been avoided or diagnosed earlier and were likely caused by incomplete polypectomy or missed cancer.[26]

Taken together, these studies highlight the fact that operator technique, including thoroughness of the examination and polypectomy completeness, is likely the most critical factor for high-quality and effective colonoscopy.

RELATION BETWEEN NON-POLYPOID COLORECTAL NEOPLASMS AND QUALITY COLONOSCOPY

The absolute contribution of NP-CRNs to interval cancers is not known and is unlikely to be defined with certainty because the characteristics of NP-CRNs are such that the possible reasons for not detecting these neoplasms overlap with several of the factors listed in **Box 2**. For example, an inadequate bowel preparation will decrease the likelihood of detecting subtle, small adenomas, particularly in the proximal colon.[2] This point is of particular relevance to NP-CRNs given the predilection of these neoplasms for a proximal colonic location and specifically for depressed (IIc) lesions given the aggressive behavior of these lesions.[27–32] Further, recognition of NP-CRNs may be dependent upon operator characteristics, such as perceptual skill or personality attributes, and suboptimal technique may increase the risk for incomplete polypectomy. Further compounding these issues is the fact that NP-CRNs are themselves heterogeneous with respect to tendency to progress to invasive malignant disease. It is now known that depressed NP-CRNs are more aggressive than flat elevated (IIa) and flat (IIb) NP-CRNs, with 22% to 59% harboring high-grade dysplasia at the time of diagnosis.[3,30,32–34] Fortunately, it appears that IIc lesions form a small proportion of NP-CRNs, and it takes several hundred colonoscopies to detect one depressed cancer in average-risk screening populations.[3,30,35] Estimating the absolute contribution of NP-CRNs to interval cancers also requires knowledge of the true prevalence of NP-CRNs in average-risk Western populations, which is not known. Studies have reported a high rate of variation in the prevalence of NP-CRNs; among all adenomas, the proportion of NP-CRNs has ranged from 7% to 54%[3,28,30–34,36,37] (**Table 1**) and this is likely because of three major factors. First, the definition of flat neoplasms has evolved over the years; The Japanese Society for Cancer of the Colon and Rectum

Table 1
Selected Western studies reporting non-polypoid colorectal neoplasms prevalence rates

Author, Year (Ref)	N	Total Number of Adenomas	Number of NP-CRNs	Percentage of Adenomas Classified as NP-CRN (%)
Hurlstone et al 2003[33]	850	733	285	39
Jaramillo et al 1995[34]	232	261	109	42
Kahi et al 2009[35]	660	780	338	43
Rembacken et al 2000[30]	1000	321	117	36
Rex and Helbig 2007[37]	434	798	430	54
Saitoh et al 2001[31]	211	139	57	41
Soetikno et al 2008[3]	1819	1535	227	15
Tsuda et al 2002[32]	371	973	66	7

defines a lesion as flat when its height (estimated visually) is less than half its diameter and the Paris classification extends this system by defining non-polypoid lesions as neoplasms that protrude less than 2.5 mm into the colon lumen (estimated during endoscopy by comparing the height of closed biopsy forceps' cups to the height of the neoplasm).[38] In practice, it is still sometimes difficult to distinguish polypoid from non-polypoid neoplasms, especially in the case of diminutive polyps (diameter <5 mm). It is also likely that a lack of familiarity of Western endoscopists with the new nomenclature and tendency to report polyps as traditional pedunculated or sessile are contributors to the variable prevalence rates. The second major factor is that the studies listed in **Table 1**[3,28,30–34,36,37] have enrolled heterogeneous populations, including patients at high risk for colorectal neoplasia. Thus, the quoted prevalence rates may not necessarily be applicable to the broader average-risk population undergoing screening colonoscopy. Third, the methods employed to enhance the detection of NP-CRNs were not standardized, with studies employing various combinations of pan-colonic chromoendoscopy, targeted chromoendoscopy, magnification, standard definition, or high-definition optics. Many studies have used white light only to detect and classify NP-CRNs; however, these neoplasms often require additional maneuvers, such as dye spraying to accurately bring out the size, shape, and presence of depression.[3]

An estimate of the true prevalence of NP-CRN can be inferred from studies that have reported the highest overall adenoma detection rates and reported the detection rate of NP-CRNs using the Paris classification system. One such study is a randomized trial of colonoscopy withdrawal in white light versus narrow-band imaging (NBI) in 434 subjects aged 50 year or older with intact.[37] There was no significant difference in the proportions of subjects with at least one adenoma (white light 67% vs NBI 65%, $P = .61$) or in the subset of 257 subjects undergoing screening (58% vs 57%; $P = .91$). In subjects undergoing screening colonoscopy, there were 1.4 ± 1.8 adenomas per colonoscopy in the white light arm compared with 1.7 ± 2.5 in the NBI arm ($P = .73$); the rates for flat adenomas were 0.7 ± 1.1 and 0.8 ± 1.3, respectively ($P = .85$). In this study, the prevalence of adenomas was the highest reported in colonoscopy studies and was mostly accounted for by detection of large numbers of adenomas, including flat adenomas less than or equal to 5 mm in diameter.[37] In another randomized trial of high-definition pan-colonic indigo carmine chromocolonoscopy compared with high-definition white light colonoscopy, a total of 1713 polyps were found and resected in 660 average-risk subjects undergoing their first screening colonoscopy. Of these, 780 (45.5%) were adenomas, of which 35 (4.5%) were advanced adenomas. A total of 899 (52%) polyps were classified as flat according to the Paris classification, of which 338 (38%) were adenomas. Overall, the mean number of adenomas per subject was 1.2 ± 2.1, the mean number of flat polyps per subject was 1.4 ± 1.9, and the mean number of flat adenomas per subject was 0.5 ± 1.0.[36] Overall, these studies suggest that at least 40% of adenomas can be classified as non-polypoid in average-risk populations. The contribution of these neoplasms to interval cancers is not known with certainty; however, about half of interval cancers are caused by missed or incompletely removed neoplasms. Given the prevalence rate of depressed NP-CRNs (1 in 100 to 1 in 250),[3,30] it is conceivable that these neoplasms account for a significant proportion of interval cancers, at least in studies reporting the highest incidence rates.[14–16]

As previously discussed, the minimum adenoma detection rates in healthy asymptomatic patients aged 50 years or older who are undergoing screening colonoscopy are 25% for men and 15% for women; however, there is accumulating evidence that these rates underestimate the true prevalence of adenomas in average-risk screening populations. Given that studies have now established that NP-CRNs are prevalent in Western populations, and the fact that NP-CRNs have characteristics that render them exquisitely sensitive to the level of quality with which colonoscopy is performed, it is reasonable to consider that improved detection of NP-CRNs will be reflected in improved overall adenoma detection rates, reflecting more thorough and higher-quality colonoscopies. These considerations are contingent on additional studies to define the true prevalence rate of NP-CRNs in average-risk patients, and to assess the interobserver variability among colonoscopists using the same polyp classification system, such as the Paris system.

REFERENCES

1. Levin B, Lieberman DA, McFarland B, et al. Screening and surveillance for the early detection of colorectal cancer and adenomatous polyps, 2008: a joint guideline from the American Cancer Society, the US Multi-Society Task Force on Colorectal Cancer, and the American College of Radiology. CA Cancer J Clin 2008;58(3):130–60.
2. Rex DK. Maximizing detection of adenomas and cancers during colonoscopy. Am J Gastroenterol 2006;101(12):2866–77.
3. Soetikno RM, Kaltenbach T, Rouse RV, et al. Prevalence of non-polypoid (flat and depressed) colorectal neoplasms in asymptomatic and symptomatic adults. JAMA 2008;299(9):1027–35.
4. Rex DK, Petrini JL, Baron TH, et al. Quality indicators for colonoscopy. Gastrointest Endosc 2006;63(Suppl 4):S16–28.
5. Harewood GC, Sharma VK, de Garmo P. Impact of colonoscopy preparation quality on detection of suspected colonic neoplasia. Gastrointest Endosc 2003; 58(1):76–9.
6. Froehlich F, Wietlisbach V, Gonvers JJ, et al. Impact of colonic cleansing on quality and diagnostic yield of colonoscopy: the European panel of appropriateness of Gastrointestinal Endoscopy European Multicenter Study. Gastrointest Endosc 2005;61(3):378–84.
7. Parra-Blanco A, Nicolas-Perez D, Gimeno-Garcia A, et al. The timing of bowel preparation before colonoscopy determines the quality of cleansing, and is a significant factor contributing to the detection of flat lesions: a randomized study. World J Gastroenterol 2006;12(38):6161–6.
8. Harewood GC, Chrysostomou K, Himy N, et al. Impact of operator fatigue on endoscopy performance: implications for procedure scheduling. Dig Dis Sci 2009;54(8):1656–61.
9. Sanaka MR, Deepinder F, Thota PN, et al. Adenomas are detected more often in morning than in afternoon colonoscopy. Am J Gastroenterol 2009;104(7):1659–64 [quiz: 1665].
10. Barclay RL, Vicari JJ, Doughty AS, et al. Colonoscopic withdrawal times and adenoma detection during screening colonoscopy. N Engl J Med 2006; 355(24):2533–41.
11. Winawer SJ, Zauber AG, Ho MN, et al. Prevention of colorectal cancer by colonoscopic polypectomy. The National Polyp Study Workgroup. N Engl J Med 1993; 329(27):1977–81.
12. Zauber A, Winawer SJ, O'brien MJ, et al. Significant long term reduction in colorectal cancer mortality with colonoscopic polypectomy: findings of the National Polyp Study. Gastroenterology 2007;132:A50.

13. Citarda F, Tomaselli G, Capocaccia R, et al. Efficacy in standard clinical practice of colonoscopic polypectomy in reducing colorectal cancer incidence. Gut 2001; 48(6):812–5.

14. Alberts DS, Martinez ME, Roe DJ, et al. Lack of effect of a high-fiber cereal supplement on the recurrence of colorectal adenomas. Phoenix Colon Cancer Prevention Physicians' Network. N Engl J Med 2000;342(16):1156–62.

15. Schatzkin A, Lanza E, Corle D, et al. Lack of effect of a low-fat, high-fiber diet on the recurrence of colorectal adenomas. Polyp Prevention Trial Study Group. N Engl J Med 2000;342(16):1149–55.

16. Robertson DJ, Greenberg ER, Beach M, et al. Colorectal cancer in patients under close colonoscopic surveillance. Gastroenterology 2005;129(1):34–41.

17. Brenner H, Chang-Claude J, Seiler CM, et al. Does a negative screening colonoscopy ever need to be repeated? Gut 2006;55(8):1145–50.

18. Singh H, Turner D, Xue L, et al. Risk of developing colorectal cancer following a negative colonoscopy examination: evidence for a 10-year interval between colonoscopies. JAMA 2006;295(20):2366–73.

19. Singh G, Gerson L, Wang H, et al. Screening colonoscopy, colorectal cancer and gender: an unfair deal for the fair sex? Gastrointest Endosc 2007;65:AB100.

20. Baxter NN, Goldwasser MA, Paszat LF, et al. Association of colonoscopy and death from colorectal cancer. Ann Intern Med 2009;150(1):1–8.

21. Arain MA, Sawhney M, Sheikh S, et al. CIMP status of interval colon cancers: another piece to the puzzle. Am J Gastroenterol 2010;105(5):1189–95.

22. Sawhney MS, Farrar WD, Gudiseva S, et al. Microsatellite instability in interval colon cancers. Gastroenterology 2006;131(6):1700–5.

23. DeVault KR, D'Alessandro AD, Albright JB, et al. Development of colon cancer while in a screening and surveillance program. Am J Gastroenterol 2007;102: S259.

24. Farrar WD, Sawhney MS, Nelson DB, et al. Colorectal cancers found after a complete colonoscopy. Clin Gastroenterol Hepatol 2006;4(10):1259–64.

25. Bressler B, Paszat LF, Chen Z, et al. Rates of new or missed colorectal cancers after colonoscopy and their risk factors: a population-based analysis. Gastroenterology 2007;132(1):96–102.

26. Pabby A, Schoen RE, Weissfeld JL, et al. Analysis of colorectal cancer occurrence during surveillance colonoscopy in the dietary polyp prevention trial. Gastrointest Endosc 2005;61(3):385–91.

27. Brooker JC, Saunders BP, Shah SG, et al. Total colonic dye-spray increases the detection of diminutive adenomas during routine colonoscopy: a randomized controlled trial. Gastrointest Endosc 2002;56(3):333–8.

28. Hurlstone DP, Cross SS, Slater R, et al. Detecting diminutive colorectal lesions at colonoscopy: a randomised controlled trial of pan-colonic versus targeted chromoscopy. Gut 2004;53(3):376–80.

29. Kiesslich R, von Bergh M, Hahn M, et al. Chromoendoscopy with indigocarmine improves the detection of adenomatous and nonadenomatous lesions in the colon. Endoscopy 2001;33(12):1001–6.

30. Rembacken BJ, Fujii T, Cairns A, et al. Flat and depressed colonic neoplasms: a prospective study of 1000 colonoscopies in the UK. Lancet 2000;355(9211): 1211–4.

31. Saitoh Y, Waxman I, West AB, et al. Prevalence and distinctive biologic features of flat colorectal adenomas in a North American population. Gastroenterology 2001; 120(7):1657–65.

32. Tsuda S, Veress B, Toth E, et al. Flat and depressed colorectal tumours in a southern Swedish population: a prospective chromoendoscopic and histopathological study. Gut 2002;51(4):550–5.
33. Hurlstone DP, Cross SS, Adam I, et al. A prospective clinicopathological and endoscopic evaluation of flat and depressed colorectal lesions in the United Kingdom. Am J Gastroenterol 2003;98(11):2543–9.
34. Jaramillo E, Watanabe M, Slezak P, et al. Flat neoplastic lesions of the colon and rectum detected by high-resolution video endoscopy and chromoscopy. Gastrointest Endosc 1995;42(2):114–22.
35. Kahi CJ, Imperiale TF, Juliar BE, et al. Effect of screening colonoscopy on colorectal cancer incidence and mortality. Clin Gastroenterol Hepatol 2009;7(7):770–5 [quiz: 711].
36. Kahi CJ, Anderson J, Waxman I, et al. High-definition chromocolonoscopy versus high-definition white light colonoscopy for average-risk colorectal cancer screening. Am J Gastroenterol 2010. [Epub ahead of print]. DOI:10.1038/ajg.2009.699.
37. Rex DK, Helbig CC. High yields of small and flat adenomas with high-definition colonoscopes using either white light or narrow band imaging. Gastroenterology 2007;133(1):42–7.
38. The Paris endoscopic classification system of superficial neoplastic lesions: esophagus, stomach, and colon. Gastrointest Endosc 2003;58(Suppl 6):S3–43.

Non-Polypoid Colorectal Neoplasms are Relatively Common Worldwide

Ana Ignjatovic, BA, BMBCh, MRCP, Brian P. Saunders, MD, FRCP*

KEYWORDS

• Polyps • Neoplasms • Non-polypoid • Prevalence

Polypoid adenomas are considered to be the precursors of most sporadic colorectal cancers (CRCs), following the adenoma-carcinoma sequence.[1,2] However, up to 10% of CRCs detected at colonoscopy are small (<1.5 cm), flat lesions with little or no adenomatous component[3–7] and an alternative hypothesis of CRC oncogenesis has been proposed characterized by relatively rapid progression from flat adenoma to invasive cancer. Flat adenomas may in fact be the precursors of the vast majority of ulcerating cancers, particularly in the proximal colon; therefore, identification and complete excision of flat adenomas is a crucial part of effective cancer prevention.

The term "flat adenoma" was first used by Muto[8] in 1985 to describe 33 flat elevated lesions smaller than 1 cm, detected at colonoscopy or in surgically resected specimens. This article was considered largely irrelevant in the West, as flat adenomas were thought to be exclusively a Japanese phenomenon. However, with Japanese endoscopists traveling to many western centers and encouraging western colleagues to adopt careful examination technique, flat adenomas have now been described worldwide, albeit with widely varying prevalence. This is probably attributable to a combination of factors, including case-mix; geographic variation; quality of colonoscopy, both in terms of individual colonoscopist and the equipment used (degree of definition and advanced imaging); and the lack of standardized endoscopic and histologic definitions. The Paris endoscopic classification has been a major step forward in defining superficial neoplastic lesions.[9] Flat adenomas are therefore described as superficial, non-polypoid colorectal neoplasia (NP-CRN) and can be slightly elevated (0–IIa), flush with the mucosa, ie, truly flat (0–IIb), slightly depressed (0–IIc), or a combination of elevation with central depression and vice versa (0–IIa+IIc; 0–IIc+IIa). Those with a depression (true IIc component) are thought to be of particular biologic

Wolfson Unit for Endoscopy, Imperial College, St Mark's Hospital, Watford Road, Harrow, HA1 3UJ, London, UK
* Corresponding author.
E-mail address: b.saunders@imperial.ac.uk

Gastrointest Endoscopy Clin N Am 20 (2010) 417–429
doi:10.1016/j.giec.2010.03.002
1052-5157/10/$ – see front matter © 2010 Elsevier Inc. All rights reserved.

significance and are more likely to harbor higher grade dysplasia or submucosal cancer[10] when compared with flat elevated or polypoid lesions of the same size.

WORLDWIDE PREVALENCE OF NP-CRN
Data from Asia

Early Japanese studies (**Table 1**) suggested that NP-CRNs are relatively common. In the largest single-center series from Japan, Kudo and Kashida[11] reported that of 21,262 neoplastic lesions resected over a period of 19 years, 43% were non-polypoid. Similarly, a high proportion of NP-CRN (48%) was described in a recent study from Malaysia, where Rajendra and colleagues[12] prospectively studied the prevalence of flat colonic adenomas, defined as mucosal elevations with height less than half of the diameter of the lesion. A lower proportion of NP-CRN was demonstrated, however, in 2 retrospective pathologic studies from Japan. Kubota and colleagues[13] examined 297 adenomas obtained from 300 surgically resected colons and found that 57 adenomas (19%) could be classified as flat (defined as having a flat surface) or depressed lesions. Similarly, Ajioka and colleagues[14] reported that 140 (22%) of 643 adenomas could be described as having non-polypoid morphology (≤ 3 mm in height). Two prospective colonoscopy studies from Korea found a significantly lower frequency of NP-CRN. Kil Lee and colleagues[15] assessed the morphology of 3263 lesions larger than 5 mm in 1883 patients and found a 7% frequency of NP-CRN, whereas in a study of 3360 patients by Park and colleagues,[16] 6% of adenomas were considered flat.[12]

Data from Western Countries

Studies from the United Kingdom, United States, Canada, Sweden, Spain, and Germany (**Table 2**) have similarly reported very different frequencies of NP-CRN (7%–42%). Defining non-polypoid lesions as those where the diameter is several times greater than the height of the lesion, Jaramillo and colleagues[17] detected 261 polyps in 178 patients, 109 (42%) of which were flat. Two prospective studies from the United Kingdom[18,19] reported a frequency of flat (lesion height > half the diameter) and depressed adenomas as 37% and 41% respectively. Much lower rates have been reported from Canada[20] (9%) and Sweden[21] (7%) but both of these studies were retrospective and required a histologic definition of flat adenoma (the height of adenoma was > half of the adjacent normal mucosa), which may account for differences observed. In the United States, Soetikno and colleagues[22] prospectively studied prevalence of NP-CRN in 1819 predominantly white, male patients undergoing screening (34%), surveillance (36%), or diagnostic colonoscopy (30%). NP-CRNs were detected in 170 (9.35%) patients and represented 15% of all adenomas detected. Prevalence of NP-CRN varied according to the indication for colonoscopy (screening 5.84%, surveillance 15.44%, and symptoms 6.01%). These findings are similar to those reported by an earlier small prospective study of 148 patients from Nebraska.[23] Prevalence of NP-CRN was 12% overall and higher (17%) in those patients with previous history of colonic neoplasia. In this study, flat adenomas were found in similar proportions in patients younger and older than 61, unlike polypoid adenomas, which were significantly more common in the older age group.

REASONS FOR VARIATION IN WORLDWIDE PREVALENCE OF NP ADENOMAS

This literature review, which spans the past 2 decades of endoscopy research, has highlighted that NP-CRNs are found throughout the world, but the definitions of what constitutes flat CRN are highly variable. In 2000, the Paris Workshop[9] attempted to standardize the terminology of superficial colorectal neoplasia; however, even studies published since then have used a number of different, often vague definitions. A number of other factors have contributed to different frequencies and prevalence of NP-CRN reported by different groups. Over the past 25 years, there have been dramatic changes in endoscopic technology and technique, which have had an impact on detection rates of all lesions but particularly those with subtle morphologic changes such as flat adenomas. Most recent studies from the East or West have incorporated both high-definition endoscopes and optimal examination technique with a corresponding higher prevalence of flat lesion detection. Expertise of the colonoscopist performing the procedure and his or her awareness of small, non-polypoid lesions is clearly important for detection. When a Japanese expert trained in flat lesion detection and an American colonoscopist examined 211 American patients in a single center, 23% were found to have non-polypoid lesions. This group was compared with a control group of patients who underwent colonoscopy performed only by the American gastroenterologist where significantly fewer lesions of any kind were found and particularly polyps smaller than 5 mm. Enhancing mucosal contrast, either by using a dye or advanced optical imaging, may improve the detection of subtle, flat lesions. Chromoendoscopy with indigocarmine increases detection of flat or depressed CRN.[24–27] Using targeted chromoendoscopy when a non-polypoid lesion was suspected, Rubio and colleagues[28] detected 109 flat adenomas in 55 (24%) of 232 patients. This is similar to the findings of Saitoh and colleagues[29] where, by using chromoscopy routinely in the left colon and targeted use of dye to any suspicious lesions in the right colon, they detected NP-CRN in 48 (23%) patients. Although narrow-band imaging (NBI) does not improve overall adenoma detection, it may be helpful when examining for non-polypoid lesions.[30,31] East and colleagues[30] examined 62 patients from HNPCC families attending for colonoscopic surveillance, first with white light colonoscopy then with NBI in a back-to-back study design. The proportion of flat adenomas detected with NBI was significantly higher than that detected with white light (45% vs 12%, $P = .03$).

BIOLOGIC SIGNIFICANCE OF NP-CRN

There is a long-standing debate about the biologic significance of flat adenomas ever since Muto's initial paper where 40% of flat lesions contained high-grade dysplasia (**Table 3**).[32] In this study, however, all lesions were described as depressed and later data by Muto and colleagues[33] suggest that the prevalence of high-grade dysplasia in all small flat adenomas is much lower, at 13%. Other Japanese investigators have similarly reported a higher prevalence of high-grade dysplasia and early submucosally invasive cancer in flat-depressed compared with flat-elevated lesions. Adachi and colleagues[10] reported that central depression was observed in 19% of 236 flat adenomas resected from 183 patients. The rate of severe atypia of flat adenomas with central depression (22%) was significantly higher than that of flat adenomas without central depression (9%; $P<.05$). Furthermore, in a series published by Kudo and Kashida,[11] 33% of depressed lesions demonstrated submucosal invasion (T1 cancer) compared with 1% of flat elevated and 2% of protruded lesions.

Early studies from the United States, which failed to separate histology findings for flat depressed polyps versus flat elevated polyps, did not support the idea that flat polyps were more likely to contain high-grade dysplasia (HGD) or cancer when compared with protruded polyps.[23,34] When sessile adenomas from the National Polyp Study cohort[35] were reclassified histologically as flat or polypoid, 27% of adenomas were reclassified as flat (adenoma thickness <1.3 mm); however, flat

Table 1
Prevalence of NP-CRN in the East (excludes cancer unless indicated)

Study	Year	No. of Patients Studied	No. of Patients with NP-CRN (% of All Patients)	Overall no. of Adenomas	No. of NP-CRN (% of All Adenomas Detected)	No. of NP-CRN with Depressed Morphology (% of flat adenomas)
Matsumoto et al[43]	1992	—	32 / —	—	34[b] / —	26 (76%)
Kudo[44]	1993	—	— / —	563	225 (40%)	99 (44%)
Karita et al[45,d]	1993	—	29 / —	—	27 / —	—
Matsumoto et al[39]	1994	895	36 (4%)[a]	634	34 (5%)	—
Minamoto et al[46]	1994	—	— / —	—	17 / —	6 (35%)
Mitooka et al[47]	1995	1152	32 (3%)	—	37[b] / —	28 (76%)
Kubota et al[13]	1996	—	— / —	297	57 (19%)	25 (44%)

Kudo et al[48]	2000	—	—	13,718	6097 (44%)	229 (4%)
Ajioka et al[14]	2000	—	—	643	140 (22%)	40 (29%)
Rajendra et al[12,d]	2003	426	7 (2%)c	29	14 (48%)	—
Kudo and Kashida[11,d]	2005	—	—	21,262	9189 (43%)	505 (5%)
Park et al[16,d]	2008	3360	207 (6%)c	—	—	—
LeeKil Lee et al[15,d]	2008	1883	189 (10%)	3128	228 (7%)	—

a Includes 8 cancers.
b Polyps <5 mm only.
c Polyps ≥5 mm only.
d Prospective studies.

Table 2
Prevalence of NP-CRN in the West (excludes cancer unless indicated)

Study	Year	No. of Patients Studied	No. of Patients with NP-CRN (% of All Patients)	Overall no. of Adenomas	No. of NP-CRN (% of All Adenomas Detected)	No. of NP-CRN with Depressed Morphology (% of Flat Adenomas)
Wolber and Owen[20] (Canada)	1991	210	18 (9%)	340	29 (9%)	—
Lanspa et al[23,a] (USA)	1992	148	18 (12%)	66	—	—
Jaramillo et al[38,a] (Sweden)	1995	232	55 (24%)	261	109 (42%)	14 (13%)
Fujii et al[18,a] (UK)	1998	210	—	68	28 (41%)	2 (7%)
Rembacken et al[19,a] (UK)	2000	1000	—	321	119 (37%)	2 (2%)
Saitoh et al[29,a] (USA)	2001	211	48 (23%)	136	54 (40%)	—
Kiesslich et al[26,a] (Germany)	2001	100	—	26	5 (19%)	1 (25%)

Study	Year	No. of patients	Depressed type n (%)	Total NP lesions	NP adenoma n (%)	NP cancer n (%)
Tsuda et al[21,a] (Sweden)	2002	866	52 (6%)	957	61 (7%)	14 (23%)
Hurlstone et al[49,a] (UK)	2003	850	—	733	267 (36%)	41 (15%)
O'Brien et al[36] (USA)	2004	938	335 (36%)	1750	474 (27%)	—
Diebold et al[50,a,b] (France)	2004	196	—	173	65 (38%)	—
Suzuki et al[51] (UK)	2006	500	—	330	63 (19%)	7 (11%)
Parra-Blanco et al[52] (Spain)	2006	1105	—	490	114 (23%)	3 (3%)
Soetikno et al[22,a] (USA)	2008	1819	170 (9%)	1523	223 (15%)	16 (7%)
Gorgun and Church[53] (USA)	2009	2659	212 (11%)	3115	338 (11%)	23 (7%)

[a] Prospective studies.
[b] Polyps >3 mm only.

Table 3
High-grade dysplasia and cancer in NP-CRN

Study	NP-CRN/ Overall CRN (%)	No. of NP-CRN with HGD (% of All NP-CRN)	No. of NP-CRN with at Least T1 Carcinoma (% of All NP-CRN)	No. of Depressed Lesions (% of All NP-CRN)	No. of Depressed NP-CRN with HGD (% of All Depressed Lesions)	No. of Depressed NP-CRN with T1 Carcinoma (% of All Depressed Lesions)
Muto et al 1985[8]	33 —	14 (42%)	0 (0%)	33 —	14 (42%)	0 —
Jaramillo et al 1994[17]	109 (42%)	13 (12%)	3 (3%)	—	—	0 —
Wolber and Owen 1991[20]	29 (9%)	12 (41%)	—	—	—	—
Karita et al 1993[45]	27 —	13 (48%)	0 (0%)	—	—	—
Minamoto et al 1994[46]	26 —	7 (27%)	5 (19%)	10 (38%)	4 (40%)	1 (10%)
Mitooka et al 1995[47]	—	14%	0	76%	18%	0
Rubio et al 1995[28]	287 —	16 (15%)	3 (3%)	—	—	—
Adachi et al 2000[10]	236 —	28 (12%)	0	46 (19%)	10 (22%)	0 (0%)
Fujii et al 1998[18]	28 (41%)	1 (4%)	2 (7%)	3 (11%)	1 (33%)	2 (66%)

Study						
Kudo et al 2000[19]	6231 (44%)	—	134 (2%)	325 (5%)	—	96 (30%)
Rembacken et al 2000[19]	123 (37%)	16 (13%)	4 (3%)	4 (3%)	1 (25%)	2 (50%)
Kiesslich et al 2001[26]	6 (19%)	2 (33%)	1 (17%)	2 (33%)	1 (50%)	1 (50%)
Saitoh et al 2001[29]	57 (41%)	—	3 (5%)	—	—	—
Tsuda et al 2002[21]	66 (7%)	11 (18%)	5 (8%)	18 (27%)	1 (6%)	4 (22%)
Hurlstone et al 2003[49]	285 (39%)	66 (23%)	18 (6%)	51 (18%)	30 (59%)	18 (35%)
Kudo and Kashida 2005[11]	9189 (43%)	—	263 (3%)	505 (5%)	—	166 (33%)
Park et al 2008[16,b]	207 (6%)	8 (4%)	3ᵃ (1%)	—	—	—
Kil Lee et al 2008[15,b]	254 (8%)	24 (9%)	26ᵃ (10%)	—	—	—
Soetikno et al 2008[22]	227 (15%)	—	15ᵃ (7%)	18 (8%)	—	6ᵃ (33%)

Abbreviation: HGD, high-grade dysplasia.
ᵃ Includes carcinoma in situ.
ᵇ Polyps ≥5 mm only.

adenomas were no more likely to contain HGD than polypoid ones, when corrected for size, location, and villous components.[36] However, later studies from the West that separated NP-CRN into depressed and flat elevated lesions confirmed Japanese findings that the presence of a depressed element is a particularly sinister prognostic indicator in flat lesions. A Swedish study[21] found the rate of high-grade dysplasia was more frequently found in flat elevated adenomas with central depression (IIa+IIc) and depressed (IIc) adenomas (36%) than in flat elevated adenomas (IIa) (13%).

Lesions containing a type IIc NP-CRN component are also associated with a higher frequency of carcinoma, although prevalence varies between East and West. This may be mainly because of lack of a uniform histopathological definition for cancer. Japanese histopathologists diagnose cancer on the basis of cellular atypia and not on the degree of penetration through muscularis mucosae as is the case in the West (World Health Organization definition).[37] When an experienced Japanese endoscopist examined 210 consecutive British patients using chromoendoscopy to highlight any subtle abnormalities, 38% of adenomas found were flat and 3% were depressed. Of 7 lesions that had severe dysplasia or invasive cancer, 4 (57%) had an area of central depression. Conversely, flat elevated lesions without depression mostly contained low-grade dysplasia. Rembacken and colleagues[19] in their study of 1000 colonoscopies found 321 adenomas of which 36% were flat and 0.6% depressed. Polyps smaller than 10 mm, whether polypoid or flat, were unlikely to contain early cancer, but 29% of flat lesions 10 mm or larger and 75% of all depressed lesions contained early cancer. These findings were confirmed by studies from the United States. Soetikno and colleagues[22] reported that non-polypoid lesions were more likely to contain carcinoma regardless of size (odds ratio 9.78; 95% confidence interval 3.93–24.40). Although flat and depressed lesions represented only 15% of all neoplasms, 54% of all superficial cancers (defined as intramucosal and T1 cancers) had non-polypoid morphology.

PREVALENCE OF FLAT CANCERS

Worldwide, the reported prevalence of flat cancers at colonoscopy ranges from 0.1% to 0.9%.[5,19,38,39] Histologically, 44% to 100% of small, flat cancers are reported to have no adenomatous component[5,7] and may therefore develop from non-polypoid lesions.[6] A study of 2198 colonoscopies from the United Kingdom[40] demonstrated that of 18 early (T1) cancers detected, half were flat and, of those, a third were 10 mm or smaller in diameter. Similar findings were reported from another UK center by Suzuki and colleagues,[41] who retrospectively reviewed 1026 consecutive colonoscopies and found 47 cases of CRC. There were 5 NP-CRNs (mean size 11 mm), which represented 10% of all cancers and 71% of T1 lesions detected. Similarly, Ishihara and colleagues[42] found the overall incidence of small (<20 mm), flat cancer to be low at 1.3% with 65.0% having non-polypoid morphology. This suggests that the incidence and natural history of these small non-polypoid cancers is similar in the East and West.

SUMMARY

Flat adenomas are found commonly at colonoscopy throughout the world, accounting for 7% to 44% of all adenomas. Similarly, small, flat submucosally invasive cancers have been described worldwide but are relatively rare, accounting for 5% to 10% of all cancers detected at colonoscopy. Although there appears to be no difference in frequency of NP-CRN between East and West, considerable variation has been reported by individual studies, probably because of lack of consistency when defining a flat lesion; a problem that has to a greater extent now been addressed by the Paris Classification.[9] Flat elevated lesions are the most common type of flat lesion and do not appear to have a greatly increased risk of harboring invasive malignancy; however, flat lesions with depression (IIa +IIc or IIc lesions) have a significant risk of malignancy and are probably the precursor lesions for most small, flat, or ulcerating cancers.

REFERENCES

1. Morson B. President's address. The polyp-cancer sequence in the large bowel. Proc R Soc Med 1974;67(6 Pt 1):451–7.
2. Vogelstein B, Fearon ER, Hamilton SR, et al. Genetic alterations during colorectal-tumor development. N Engl J Med 1988;319(9):525–32.
3. Stolte M, Bethke B. Colorectal mini-de novo carcinoma: a reality in Germany too. Endoscopy 1995;27(4):286–90.
4. Kuramoto S, Oohara T. Flat early cancers of the large intestine. Cancer 1989; 64(4):950–5.
5. Iishi H, Tatsuta M, Tsutsui S, et al. Early depressed adenocarcinomas of the large intestine. Cancer 1992;69(10):2406–10.
6. Shimoda T, Ikegami M, Fujisaki J, et al. Early colorectal carcinoma with special reference to its development de novo. Cancer 1989;64(5):1138–46.
7. Minamoto T, Mai M, Ogino T, et al. Early invasive colorectal carcinomas metastatic to the lymph node with attention to their nonpolypoid development. Am J Gastroenterol 1993;88(7):1035–9.
8. Muto T, Kamiya J, Sawada T, et al. Small "flat adenoma" of the large bowel with special reference to its clinicopathologic features. Dis Colon Rectum 1985; 28(11):847–51.
9. The Paris endoscopic classification of superficial neoplastic lesions: esophagus, stomach, and colon: November 30 to December 1, 2002. Gastrointest Endosc 2003;58:S3–43 Paris Workshop Participants.
10. Adachi M, Okinaga K, Muto T. Flat adenoma of the large bowel: re-evaluation with special reference to central depression. Dis Colon Rectum 2000;43(6): 782–7.
11. Kudo SE, Kashida H. Flat and depressed lesions of the colorectum. Clin Gastroenterol Hepatol 2005;3(7 Suppl 1):S33–6.
12. Rajendra S, Kutty K, Karim N. Flat colonic adenomas in Malaysia: fact or fancy? J Gastroenterol Hepatol 2003;18(6):701–4.
13. Kubota O, Kino I, Kimura T, et al. Nonpolypoid adenomas and adenocarcinomas found in background mucosa of surgically resected colons. Cancer 1996;77(4): 621–6.
14. Ajioka Y, Watanabe H, Kazama S, et al. Early colorectal cancer with special reference to the superficial nonpolypoid type from a histopathologic point of view. World J Surg 2000;24(9):1075–80.
15. Kil Lee S, Kim T II, Kwan Shin S, et al. Comparison of the clinicopathologic features between flat and polypoid adenoma. Scand J Gastroenterol 2008; 43(9):1116–21.
16. Park DH, Kim HS, Kim WH, et al. Clinicopathologic characteristics and malignant potential of colorectal flat neoplasia compared with that of polypoid neoplasia. Dis Colon Rectum 2008;51(1):43–9 [discussion: 49].
17. Jaramillo E, Slezak P, Watanabe M, et al. Endoscopic detection and complete removal of a micro-invasive carcinoma present in a flat colonic adenoma. Gastrointest Endosc 1994;40(3):369–71.

18. Fujii T, Rembacken BJ, Dixon MF, et al. Flat adenomas in the United Kingdom: are treatable cancers being missed? Endoscopy 1998;30(5):437–43.
19. Rembacken BJ, Fujii T, Cairns A, et al. Flat and depressed colonic neoplasms: a prospective study of 1000 colonoscopies in the UK. Lancet 2000;355(9211): 1211–4.
20. Wolber RA, Owen DA. Flat adenomas of the colon. Hum Pathol 1991;22(1):70–4.
21. Tsuda S, Veress B, Toth E, et al. Flat and depressed colorectal tumours in a southern Swedish population: a prospective chromoendoscopic and histopathological study. Gut 2002;51(4):550–5.
22. Soetikno RM, Kaltenbach T, Rouse RV, et al. Prevalence of nonpolypoid (flat and depressed) colorectal neoplasms in asymptomatic and symptomatic adults. JAMA 2008;299(9):1027–35.
23. Lanspa SJ, Rouse J, Smyrk T, et al. Epidemiologic characteristics of the flat adenoma of Muto. A prospective study. Dis Colon Rectum 1992;35(6): 543–6.
24. Brooker JC, Saunders BP, Shah SG, et al. Total colonic dye-spray increases the detection of diminutive adenomas during routine colonoscopy: a randomized controlled trial. Gastrointest Endosc 2002;56(3):333–8.
25. Hurlstone DP, Cross SS, Slater R, et al. Detecting diminutive colorectal lesions at colonoscopy: a randomised controlled trial of pan-colonic versus targeted chromoscopy. Gut 2004;53(3):376–80.
26. Kiesslich R, von Bergh M, Hahn M, et al. Chromoendoscopy with indigocarmine improves the detection of adenomatous and nonadenomatous lesions in the colon. Endoscopy 2001;33(12):1001–6.
27. Hurlstone DP, Karajeh M, Cross SS, et al. The role of high-magnification-chromoscopic colonoscopy in hereditary nonpolyposis colorectal cancer screening: a prospective "back-to-back" endoscopic study. Am J Gastroenterol 2005; 100(10):2167–73.
28. Rubio CA, Jaramillo E, Slezak P. [Recently acquired knowledge of flat adenomas in the large intestine. Hidden precancerous changes demonstrable by endoscopy]. Lakartidningen 1995;92(24):2504–7.
29. Saitoh Y, Waxman I, West AB, et al. Prevalence and distinctive biologic features of flat colorectal adenomas in a North American population. Gastroenterology 2001; 120(7):1657–65.
30. East JE, Suzuki N, Stavrinidis M, et al. Narrow band imaging for colonoscopic surveillance in hereditary non-polyposis colorectal cancer. Gut 2008; 57(1):65–70.
31. Rex DK, Helbig CC. High yields of small and flat adenomas with high-definition colonoscopes using either white light or narrow band imaging. Gastroenterology 2007;133(1):42–7.
32. Muto T, Kamiya J, Sawada T, et al. Small "flat adenoma" of the large bowel with special reference to its clinicopathologic features. Dis Colon Rectum 1985; 28(11):847–51.
33. Muto T. Small flat adenomas. Gastrointest Endosc 1996;44(5):632.
34. Waye JD, Lewis BS, Frankel A, et al. Small colon polyps. Am J Gastroenterol 1988;83:120–2.
35. Winawer SJ, Zauber AG, Ho MN, et al. The National Polyp Study. Eur J Cancer Prev 1993;2(Suppl 2):83–7.
36. O'Brien MJ, Winawer SJ, Zauber AG, et al. Flat adenomas in the National Polyp Study: is there increased risk for high-grade dysplasia initially or during surveillance? Clin Gastroenterol Hepatol 2004;2(10):905–11.

37. Jass JR, Sobin LH. Histological typing of intestinal tumours: World Health Organisation. 2nd edition. Berlin: Springer; 1989.
38. Jaramillo E, Watanabe M, Slezak P, et al. Flat neoplastic lesions of the colon and rectum detected by high-resolution video endoscopy and chromoscopy. Gastrointest Endosc 1995;42(2):114–22.
39. Matsumoto T, Iida M, Yao T, et al. Role of nonpolypoid neoplastic lesions in the pathogenesis of colorectal cancer. Dis Colon Rectum 1994;37(5):450–5.
40. Smith GA, Oien KA, O'Dwyer PJ. Frequency of early colorectal cancer in patients undergoing colonoscopy. Br J Surg 1999;86(10):1328–31.
41. Suzuki N, Talbot IC, Saunders BP. The prevalence of small, flat colorectal cancers in a western population. Colorectal Dis 2004;6(1):15–20.
42. Ishihara S, Watanabe T, Umetani N, et al. Small advanced colorectal cancers: clinicopathological characteristics and pathogenetic origin. Jpn J Clin Oncol 2000;30(11):504–9.
43. Matsumoto T, Iida M, Kuwano Y, et al. Minute non-polypoid adenoma of the colon detected by colonoscopy: correlation between endoscopic and histologic findings. Gastrointest Endosc 1992;38(6):645–50.
44. Kudo S. Endoscopic mucosal resection of flat and depressed types of early colorectal cancer. Endoscopy 1993;25(7):455–61.
45. Karita M, Cantero D, Okita K. Endoscopic diagnosis and resection treatment for flat adenoma with severe dysplasia. Am J Gastroenterol 1993;88(9):1421–3.
46. Minamoto T, Sawaguchi K, Ohta T, et al. Superficial-type adenomas and adenocarcinomas of the colon and rectum: a comparative morphological study. Gastroenterology 1994;106(6):1436–43.
47. Mitooka H, Fujimori T, Maeda S, et al. Minute flat depressed neoplastic lesions of the colon detected by contrast chromoscopy using an indigo carmine capsule. Gastrointest Endosc 1995;41(5):453–9.
48. Kudo S, Kashida H, Tamura T, et al. Colonoscopic diagnosis and management of nonpolypoid early colorectal cancer. World J Surg 2000;24(9):1081–90.
49. Hurlstone DP, Cross SS, Adam I, et al. A prospective clinicopathological and endoscopic evaluation of flat and depressed colorectal lesions in the United Kingdom. Am J Gastroenterol 2003;98(11):2543–9.
50. Diebold MD, Samalin E, Merle C, et al. Colonic flat neoplasia: frequency and concordance between endoscopic appearance and histological diagnosis in a French prospective series. Am J Gastroenterol 2004;99(9):1795–800.
51. Suzuki N, Price AB, Talbot IC, et al. Flat colorectal neoplasms and the impact of the revised Vienna Classification on their reporting: a case-control study in UK and Japanese patients. Scand J Gastroenterol 2006;41(7):812–9.
52. Parra-Blanco A, Gimeno-Garcia AZ, Nicolas-Perez D, et al. Risk for high-grade dysplasia or invasive carcinoma in colorectal flat adenomas in a Spanish population. Gastroenterol Hepatol 2006;29(10):602–9.
53. Gorgun E, Church J. Flat adenomas of the large bowel: a single endoscopist study. Dis Colon Rectum 2009;52(5):972–7.

The Natural History of Non-Polypoid Colorectal Neoplasms

Nozomu Kobayashi, MD[a,*], Takahisa Matsuda, MD, PhD[b],
Yasushi Sano, MD, PhD[c]

KEYWORDS

• Non-polypoid colorectal neoplasms • Depressed lesion
• De novo cancer • Colonoscopy • Natural history

The importance of non-polypoid colorectal neoplasms (NP-CRN) is now recognized throughout the world.[1–9] There is little information, however, known about the natural history of NP-CRN, perhaps because the initial reports of NP-CRN suggested that it had high risk of invasion and lymph node metastasis as compared with polypoid lesions of similar size.[10,11] Long-term follow-up of NP-CRN without resection was therefore not an accepted treatment strategy, and had been reported only based on analysis of interval neoplasms or sporadic case reports. In addition, outside Japan, many endoscopists viewed NP-CRN, especially the depressed lesion, as a uniquely Japanese phenomenon and thus, paid little attention to such lesions, limiting the data even more. This article will summarize the available data to gain some estimates of the natural history of NP-CRN.

RADIOGRAPHIC ANALYSIS

Matsui and colleagues[12] reported a retrospective analysis of a series of colorectal cancers that were missed by double-contrast barium enema examinations. They found six depressed and seven flat lesions (41%) could be retrospectively identified as antecedent lesions that gave rise to 32 advanced cancers. The authors found that all depressed lesions developed into nonprotuberant-type advanced colorectal cancers, whereas flat or polypoid lesions had a possibility to develop into either protuberant or nonprotuberant-type advanced colorectal cancers.

[a] Department of Diagnostic Imaging, Tochigi Cancer Center, 4-9-13 Yonan, Utsunomiya, Tochigi 320-0834, Japan
[b] Endoscopy Division, National Cancer Center Hospital, 5-1-1 Tsukiji, Chuo-ku, Tokyo 104-0045, Japan
[c] Gastrointestinal Center, Sano Hospital, 2-5-1 Shimizugaoka, Tarumi-ku, Kobe, Hyogo, 655-0031, Japan
* Corresponding author.
E-mail address: nkobayas@tcc.pref.tochigi.lg.jp

Gastrointest Endoscopy Clin N Am 20 (2010) 431–435
doi:10.1016/j.giec.2010.03.003
1052-5157/10/$ – see front matter © 2010 Elsevier Inc. All rights reserved.
giendo.theclinics.com

Umetani and colleagues[13] reported 11 cases of colorectal cancers that had more than two barium enema examinations that were at least 6 months apart. Five non-polypoid submucosal invasive cancers were studied; three developed from non-polypoid and two from polypoid lesions. The authors estimated tumor doubling time to evaluate the growth rate of each tumor, and suggested that NP-CRN grew slowly compared with polypoid lesion and maintained their macroscopic morphology. The data, however, are limited.

COLONOSCOPIC ANALYSIS

Matsui and colleagues[14] reported eight early colorectal cancers that were incidentally followed by colonoscopy. Thirty-five cases, including 14 NP-CRN as initial lesions, were reviewed. They found that NP-CRN progressed to submucosally invasive cancer, retaining its non-polypoid configuration, and some flat lesions developed depressed areas during their progression. Although the authors also estimated the speed of growth compared with polypoid and non-polypoid lesions, they could not conclude which type grew more rapidly.

Sato and colleagues[15] prospectively followed 12 small flat adenomas. The size of the lesions ranged from 2 to 6 mm (median 4 mm), and the observation period ranged from 11 to 26 months (median 19 months). Although eight lesions showed various changes in their shape, only two lesions demonstrated an increase in diameter of the tumor. All of the flat lesions were subsequently removed endoscopically and found to be adenomas. The authors concluded small flat adenoma did not rapidly progress, and configuration change did not indicate tumor progression or invasion.

Watari and colleagues[16] conducted prospective colonoscopic study to elucidate the natural history of NP-CRN. The authors observed 75 colorectal tumors measuring less than 1 cm in diameter in 50 patients. The average follow-up period was 22 months, and 62 lesions (83%) were NP-CRN. They concluded similar observations as those of Sato and colleagues, although they found that 40% of small non-polypoid lesions had exophytic growth with time. This finding suggested some small non-polypoid lesions follow the adenoma–carcinoma sequence the same as polypoid lesions.

THE IMPORTANCE OF THE DEPRESSED-TYPE NP-CRN

Matsuda and colleagues[17] analyzed 6638 colorectal neoplasms, excluding advanced cancers, treated in National Cancer Center Hospital, Tokyo, Japan. There were 4471 (67%) and 2167 (33%), polypoid and non-polypoid colorectal neoplasms, respectively. Among all non-polypoid lesions, there were 178 (2.7%) depressed lesions, 109 (61%) of which were diagnosed as high-grade dysplasia or submucosally invasive cancer. Among 5538 (83%) lesions that were identified as low- or high-grade dysplasia, the proportion of depressed lesions was 1.3%. On the other hand, depressed type was identified in 39% (**Table 1**) of submucosal cancers. This discrepancy may indicate of a rapid progression rate of depressed lesions into invasive cancers.

Sano and colleagues[18] described the incidence of depressed lesions among all of colorectal neoplasms, again excluding advanced cancers. Their multicenter retrospective study conducted in eight Japanese referral institutes revealed that the incidence of depressed lesions was 1.94% (1291 depressed lesions out of 66,670 neoplasms), and, in particular, 51.2% of intramucosal depressed lesions were diagnosed as high-grade dysplasia. These data also suggested that intramucosal depressed lesions showed more aggressive behavior and were perhaps more likely

Table 1
Relationship between macroscopic type and histopathological findings

	LGD	HGD	SM-Ca
Polypoid	3781 (68.3)	578 (67.9)	112 (45.0)
Flat	1688 (30.5)	260 (30.6)	41 (16.5)
Depressed	69 (1.2)	13 (1.5)	96 (38.6)
Total	5538 (83.4)	851 (12.8)	249 (3.8)

Abbreviations: HGD, high-grade dysplasia; LGD, low-grade dysplasia; SM-Ca, submucosal invasive cancer.
Data from Matsuda T, Saito Y, Hotta K, et al. Prevalence and clinicopathological features of non-polypoid colorectal neoplasms: should we pay more attention to identifying flat and depressed lesions? Dig Endosc 2010;22(Suppl 1):S57–62.

to develop into invasive cancers as compared with the polypoid lesions. The depressed type of NP-CRN appears to be pathologically and molecular biologically distinct that other types of NP-CRN.

Several authors reported that depressed-type colorectal cancer does not arise from an adenomatous polyp. This theory was called de novo carcinogenesis, and lack of K-ras mutation was thought to be a distinctive genetic feature.[10,11,19,20] Goto and colleagues[21] reported the proportion of de novo cancers among all colorectal cancers in a cohort of 14,817 Japanese populations. The authors defined de novo cancers according to both criteria: (1) the absence of adenomatous components and (2) all lateral margins of the tumor covered with normal mucosa and non-polypoid growth pattern. They concluded that 22.9% of early colorectal cancers were de novo cancers. Chen and colleagues,[22] from Taiwan, also assessed the proportion of de novo carcinomas using the Markov model, and demonstrated about 30% of colorectal cancers arising from de novo sequence.

Table 2
Description of 13 interval cancers diagnosed within 3 years of a initial colonoscopy

Number	Macroscopic Type	Size (mm)	Location	Depth of Lesion
1	Isp (semipedunculated)	13	Sigmoid	SM
2	Isp (semipedunculated)	15	Sigmoid	SM
3	Is (sessile)	8	Rectum	SM
4	Is (sessile)	10	Sigmoid	SM
5	Is (sessile)	20	Rectum	MP
6	Is (sessile)	6	Transverse	SM
7	IIa (flat)	15	Transverse	SM
8	IIa (flat)	20	Sigmoid	SM
9	IIa + IIc (depressed)	20	Cecum	SM
10	IIa + IIc (depressed)	20	Transverse	SM
11	IIa + IIc (depressed)	10	Rectum	MP
12	IIa + IIc (depressed)	6	Ascending	SM
13	IIa + IIc (depressed)	20	Sigmoid	SS

Abbreviations: MP, muscularis; SM, submucosa; SS, subserosa.
Data from Matsuda T, Fujii T, Sano Y, et al. Five-year incidence of advanced neoplasia after initial colonoscopy in Japan: a multicenter retrospective cohort study. Jpn J Clin Oncol 2009;39:435–42.

THE JAPAN POLYP STUDY

To clarify the natural history of NP-CRN, a large cohort study focused on the detection of NP-CRN is required. Matsuda and colleagues[23] reported the results of multicenter retrospective cohort study to evaluate 5-year incidence of advanced neoplasia after initial colonoscopy. The authors studied 5309 patients with a median follow-up period of 5.1 years. Endoscopists diagnosed 13 invasive cancers on follow-up within 3 years. The initial colonoscopies were performed by Japanese endoscopists who had proficient technique with chromoendoscopy to diagnose NP-CRN, and the patients had good preparation quality, taking polyethylene glycol (PEG) solution in the morning on the day of colonoscopy, Out of the 13 incident cancer cases, seven were NP-CRN, and the mean size of these lesions was less than 15 mm in diameter (**Table 2**). These data suggested that NP-CRN is responsible for interval cancers, defined as colorectal cancers diagnosed within several years of a complete colonoscopy. Much prospective data, however, are necessary to elucidate the natural history and epidemiology of these lesions. The Japan Polyp Study (JPS) is a multicenter randomized controlled trial prospectively evaluating follow-up surveillance strategy for Japanese patients after removal of all polypoid and non-polypoid neoplasms.[24] This study is intended to continue until 2011 and hopefully will provide new information on the detection and progression of NP-CRN.

SUMMARY

The natural history of NP-CRN is mostly unknown. The results of small observational studies suggest that NP-CRN lesions develop into invasive cancer with minimal size expansion. Among NP-CRN lesions, depressed lesions show more aggressive behavior and frequently develop into invasive cancers compared with polypoid lesions, regardless of their low incidence. A large prospective cohort study focused on the detection of NP-CRN is currently ongoing.

REFERENCES

1. Muto T, Kamiya J, Sawada T, et al. Small flat adenoma of the large bowel with special reference to its clinicopathologic features. Dis Colon Rectum 1985;28: 847–51.
2. Kudo S. Endoscopic mucosal resection of flat depressed type of early colorectal cancer. Endoscopy 1993;25:455–61.
3. Fujii T, Rembacken BJ, Dixon MF, et al. Flat adenomas in the United Kingdom: are treatable cancers being missed? Endoscopy 1998;30:437–43.
4. Saitoh Y, Waxman I, West AB, et al. Prevalence and distinctive biologic features of flat colorectal adenomas in a North American population. Gastroenterology 2001; 120:1657–65.
5. Tsuda S, Veress B, Toth E, et al. Flat and depressed colorectal tumours in a southern Swedish population: a prospective chromoendoscopic and histopathological study. Gut 2002;51:550–5.
6. Rembacken BJ, Fujii T, Cairns A, et al. Flat and depressed colonic neoplasms: a prospective study of 1000 colonoscopies in the UK. Lancet 2000;355:1211–4.
7. Parra-Blanco A, Gimeno-Garcia AZ, Nicolas-Perez D, et al. Risk for high-grade dysplasia or invasive carcinoma in colorectal flat adenomas in a Spanish population. Gastroenterol Hepatol 2006;29:602–9.

8. Soetikno RM, Kaltenbach T, Rouse RV, et al. Prevalence of nonpolypoid (flay and depressed) colorectal neoplasms in asymptomatic and symptomatic adults. JAMA 2008;299:1027–35.

9. Chiu HM, Lin JT, Chen CC, et al. Prevalence and characteristics of nonpolypoid colorectal neoplasm in an asymptomatic and average-risk Chinese population. Clin Gastroenterol Hepatol 2009;7:463–70.

10. Kudo S, Kashida H, Tamura T, et al. Colonoscopic diagnosis and management of nonpolypoid early colorectal cancer. World J Surg 2000;24:1081–90.

11. Shimoda T, Ikegami M, Fujisaki J, et al. Early colorectal carcinoma with special reference to its development de novo. Cancer 1989;64:1138–46.

12. Matsui T, Yao T, Iwashita A. Natural history of early colorectal cancer. World J Surg 2000;24:1022–8.

13. Umetani N, Masaki T, Watanabe T, et al. Retrospective radiographic analysis of nonpedunculated colorectal carcinomas with special reference to tumour doubling time and morphological change. Am J Gastroenterol 2000;95:1794–9.

14. Matsui T, Tsuda S, Iwashita A, et al. Retrospective endoscopic study of developmental and configurational changes of early colorectal cancer: eight cases and a review of the literature. Dig Endosc 2004;16:1–8.

15. Sato T, Konishi F, Togashi K, et al. Prospective observation of small flat tumors in the colon through colonoscopy. Dis Colon Rectum 1999;42:1457–63.

16. Watari J, Saitoh Y, Obara T, et al. Natural history of colorectal nonpolypoid adenomas: a prospective colonoscopic study and relation with cell kinetics and K-ras mutations. Am J Gastroenterol 2002;97:2109–15.

17. Matsuda T, Saito Y, Hotta K, et al. Prevalence and clinicopathological features of nonpolrypoid colorectal neoplasms: should we pay more attention to identifying flat and depressed lesions? Dig Endosc 2010;22(Suppl 1):S57–62.

18. Sano Y, Tanaka S, Teixeira CR, et al. Endoscopic detection and diagnosis of 0-IIc neoplastic colorectal lesions. Endoscopy 2005;37:261–7.

19. Fujimori T, Satonaka K, Yamamura-Idei Y, et al. Noninvolvement of ras mutations in flat colorectal adenomas and carcinomas. Int J Cancer 1994;57:51–5.

20. Kaneko K, Fujii T, Kato S, et al. Growth pattern and genetic changes of colorectal carcinoma. Jpn J Clin Oncol 1998;28:196–201.

21. Goto H, Oda Y, Murakami Y, et al. Proportion of de novo cancers among colorectal cancers in Japan. Gastroenterology 2006;131:40–6.

22. Chen CD, Yen MF, Wang WM, et al. A case-cohort study for the disease natural history of adenoma-carcinoma and de novo carcinoma and surveillance of colon and rectum after polypectomy: implication for efficacy of colonoscopy. Br J Cancer 2003;88:1866–73.

23. Matsuda T, Fujii T, Sano Y, et al. Five-year incidence of advanced neoplasia after initial colonoscopy in Japan: a multicenter retrospective cohort study. Jpn J Clin Oncol 2009;39:435–42.

24. Sano Y, Fujii T, Oda Y, et al. A multicenter randomized controlled trial designed to evaluate follow-up surveillance strategies for colorectal cancer: the Japan Polyp Study. Dig Endosc 2004;16:376–8.

Bowel Preparation and Colonoscopy Technique To Detect Non-Polypoid Colorectal Neoplasms

H.N. Kim, MD, G.S. Raju, MD*

KEYWORDS

- Colonoscopy • Non-polypoid colorectal neoplasm • Bowel
- Colon • Colon cancer screening • Colon preparation

Colonoscopy is considered the gold standard for colon cancer screening. In a recent study, however, 0.3% to 0.9% patients were reported to develop colorectal cancer within 3 years after removal of adenomas.[1,2] Some reasons for the development of interval colorectal cancers include missed or incompletely removed lesions during the initial colonoscopy. Non-polypoid colorectal neoplasms (NP-CRNs) (**Fig. 1**) are a potential contributor to the pool of missed lesions because they can be easily missed as a result of inadequate colon preparation or examination technique.[3–6]; This article discusses the methods that are useful to improve the quality of bowel preparation and examination technique.

ENDOSCOPIC RECOGNITION OF NP-CRN

Colon preparation should be absolutely clean to detect non-polypoid colorectal neoplasia because NP-CRNs, unlike the polypoid lesions that project into the lumen and can be easily identified, can hide under a thin layer of mucus or stool lining the mucosa and be easily missed. To detect the NP-CRN, excellent visualization of the vasculature and appreciation of the mucosal surface patterns (pits and grooves) of the entire colon is critical (**Fig. 2**).

Identification of the NP-CRN requires training the eye to look for surface vascular architecture of the colonic mucosa and subtle changes in the pattern of the innominate grooves. The endoscopist should be able to clearly visualize the surface microvessels, because a subtle change in the vascular network is one of the clues to identify these

Department of Gastroenterology, Hepatology, and Nutrition, The University of Texas M.D. Anderson Cancer Center, 1515 Holcombe Boulevard, Unit 1466, Houston, TX 77030, USA
* Corresponding author.
E-mail address: gsraju@mdanderson.org

Gastrointest Endoscopy Clin N Am 20 (2010) 437–448
doi:10.1016/j.giec.2010.03.005
1052-5157/10/$ – see front matter. Published by Elsevier Inc.

giendo.theclinics.com

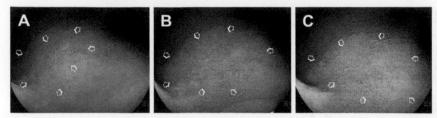

Fig. 1. A completely flat (IIb type) adenomatous lesion. Visualization of this lesion requires a completely clean colon. The lesion was examined with i-SCAN's surface enhancement feature (Pentax Medical, Montvale, NJ, USA) and showed a better delineation of the extent of lesion with higher surface enhancement. (*A*) Standard enhancement. (*B*) Medium enhancement. (*C*) High enhancement. The border of the lesion becomes more apparent with increasing enhancement—the lesion at high enhancement is larger than what is appreciated at low enhancement.

lesions. Other findings about NP-CRNs include slightly red appearance and/or friability of the mucosa and wall deformity. High-resolution endoscopy with magnification and electronic image processing (using narrow-band imaging; Fuji Intelligent Chromo Endoscopy, Fujinon Inc, Wayne, NJ, USA; or i-SCAN, Pentax of America Inc, Montvale, NJ, USA) as well as chromoendoscopy with indigo carmine may help to enhance these lesions. Interruption of the innominate grooves is another clue to the presence of subtle NP-CRN lesions.

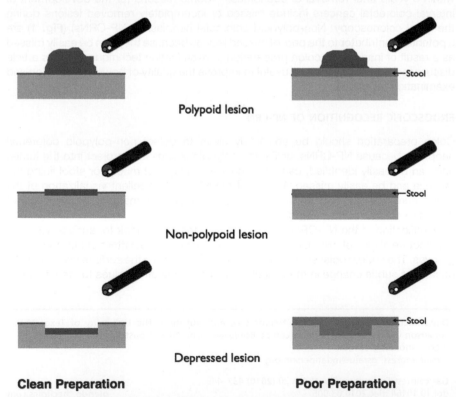

Fig. 2. Stool interferes with the detection of non-polypoid and depressed lesions.

BOWEL PREPARATION

Suboptimal bowel preparation is a significant barrier to the prevention of colon cancer with colonoscopy because[7] it results in (1) canceled procedures, (2) prolonged procedure time to clean the residual stool or mucus in the colon, and (3) missed precancerous lesions and cancer.[8-11] Of concern is the observation that bowel preparation is inadequate in almost a quarter of the patients undergoing colonoscopy in the United States.[8] The US Multi-Society Task Force on Colorectal Cancer and the American Cancer Society recommend aborting the colonoscopy when colon cleanliness is inadequate and repeating the procedure after proper preparation.[12] Two studies have recently demonstrated that the better the colon preparation, the higher is the rate of detection of precancerous lesions.[8,9] Various bowel preparation solutions, timing of the preparation, and measures useful to improve the quality of colon preparation are discussed in the following sections.

Bowel Preparation Solutions

Polyethylene glycol–based electrolyte solutions (PEG-ESLs) are the main constituents of the regimen for bowel preparation[13] (**Table 1**), given the recent Food and Drug Administration alert of acute phosphate nephropathy with sodium phosphate preparation. PEG-ESL consists of nonabsorbable, nonfermentable high-molecular-weight polymer in a dilute electrolyte solution. The solution is isosmotic, works primarily by mechanical effect of large-volume lavage, and results in minimal alteration in the balance of electrolytes and fluids.

PEG-ESL is generally well tolerated, although 5% to 15% of the patients may not complete the preparation because of poor palatability and/or large volume. A sulfate-free PEG preparation (SF-PEG), which contains less potassium and more chloride and is completely free of sodium sulfate, has been developed to improve the palatability (see **Table 1**). However, studies have failed to demonstrate that SF-PEG is better tolerated than PEG-ESL. Although flavors have been added in an attempt to improve the taste of PEG-ESL and SF-PEG, data on whether the addition of flavors has improved patient tolerance are conflicting.[14,15]

The traditionally recommended dose for an adult is 4 L taken orally: 240 mL is taken every 10 minutes until the 4 L are consumed or until the rectal output is clear. However, because of the large amount of fluid, patients frequently experience bloating, abdominal cramping, nausea, and vomiting. To address this issue, low-volume PEG-ESL preparation regimens were introduced. The total dose is 2 L, but to maintain the same efficacy, bisacodyl and magnesium citrate are usually added.

Recently the efficacies of low-volume preparations using sodium sulfate solution in lieu of sodium phosphate have been investigated. Preliminary studies report that they are effective for colon cleansing and have an acceptable safety profile. It should be noted that nonabsorbable carbohydrates such as lactulose and sorbitol have been associated with bowel explosion during electrocautery and should not be used for colon preparation.

Assessment of Bowel Preparation

The amount of residual fluid and stools in the colon is generally used to rate the quality of colon preparation. In clinical trials, terms such as "excellent," "good," "fair," and "poor" are commonly used to characterize bowel preparation quality.[16] Excellent refers to no or minimal amounts of solid stool and only small amounts of clear fluid that requires suctioning, good denotes no or minimal presence of solid stool with large amounts of clear fluid that requires suctioning, fair is when there are collections of

Table 1
PEG-based electrolyte solutions

Active Agent	Product and Manufacturer	Quantity
PEG	Colyte (Schwarz Pharma Inc, Milwaukee, WI, USA), flavored/nonflavored	4 L
PEG	GoLYTELY (Braintree Laboratories Inc, Braintree, MA, USA), flavored/nonflavored	4 L
PEG (sulfate free)	NuLYTELY (Braintree Laboratories Inc, Braintree, MA, USA), flavored/nonflavored	4 L
PEG (sulfate free)	TryLyte (Schwarz Pharma Inc, Milwaukee, WI, USA), flavored	4 L
PEG and bisacodyl	Halflytely (Braintree Laboratories Inc, Braintree, MA, USA)	PEG (2 L) and 4 bisacodyl delayed-release tablets
PEG and ascorbic acid	MoviPrep (Salix Pharmaceuticals Inc, Morrisville, NC, USA)	PEG (2 L) with ascorbic acid

semisolid debris that are cleared with difficulty, and poor refers to the presence of solid or semisolid debris that cannot be effectively cleared. However, usually, these terms do not have standardized definitions in clinical practice and their definitions depend on the endoscopist's impression. Few bowel-preparation assessment scales have been validated, and these scales have been primarily designed to compare the efficacy of different bowel preparations before any cleansing maneuvers. However, the most important aspect of rating the quality of bowel preparation is not the amount of residual colonic-lumen contents but the amount of the mucosa clearly visible for screening after cleansing maneuvers. It is not uncommon to find stool debris in the colon that can be either suctioned or moved away with water irrigation, giving an excellent view of the colon mucosa.

Recently the Boston Bowel Preparation Scale (BBPS, **Table 2**) was developed to quantify the degree of colon mucosa that can be visualized for screening after endoscopic cleansing maneuvers. This scale is more relevant for daily practice because it helps to define the subsequent plan for the patient. In addition, this new scale allows the evaluation of different segments of the colon. The colon is divided into 3 segments: right (cecum and ascending colon), transverse, and left colon (descending, sigmoid colon, and rectum), and each section is given a score of 0 to 3. A score of 0 is given when there are solid stools in the lumen, and a score of 3 when the mucosa is free of any stool or mucus. The ideal colon preparation is given a score of 9 on 9.[17] The authors have incorporated this scale in reporting the quality of colon preparation in their practice and it helps to decide better the timing of the repeat procedure (see **Table 2**).

Measures to Improve Bowel Preparation

Split-dose regimen

Several studies have shown that a split dose of PEG-ESL, in which half of the dose is consumed during the night before and the other half is consumed during the morning of the procedure, is more effective in cleaning the colon than a single dose consumed the evening before the procedure.[18–21] The morning dose in the split-dose regimen acts likes a final rinse (after the wash with the evening dose) to clear all the gastrointestinal and pancreatobiliary secretions that enter the colon during the night.[22] This

Table 2		
Boston Bowel Preparation Scale (BBPS)		
Score	Description	
0	Unprepared colon segment with mucosa not seen because of solid stool that cannot be cleared	
1	Portion of mucosa of the colon segment seen, but other areas of the colon segment are not well seen because of staining, residual stool, and/or opaque liquid	
2	Minor amount of residual staining, small fragments of stool, and/or opaque liquid, but mucosa of colon segment is seen well	
3	Entire mucosa of colon segment seen well with no residual staining, small fragments of stool, or opaque liquid	

The right, transverse, and left colons are scored from 0 to 3, and these segment scores are summed for a total BBPS score.
Data from Lai EJ, Calderwood AH, Doros G, et al. The Boston bowel preparation scale: a valid and reliable instrument for colonoscopy-oriented research. Gastrointest Endosc 2009; 69(3 Suppl):620–5.

final rinse with the morning dose is critical for detection of the flat and depressed lesions.

Although there are concerns about disruption of the sleep and travel to the endoscopy unit with the use of split dosing, both dosing schedules (single overnight and split dose) cause similar degree of disruption.[23] In their practice, the authors have observed that the patients prefer to take the morning dose to avoid the consequences of a poor preparation and repeat colonoscopy. Proper education about the benefits of the split dose results in better patient compliance and better preparation.

Timing of the split dose
In addition to the split dose, another important variable in the colon preparation for colonoscopy is the time interval between the consumption of the last dose of PEG-ESL and the procedure. An interval of 5 to 8 hours between the last dose and the colonoscopy provided the best bowel cleansing, whereas an interval of more than 14 hours resulted in a poor quality of cleansing.[24] Therefore, patients scheduled for colonoscopy before noon should take the PEG-ESL in the early hours of the morning.

Most patients would be willing to wake up and take the second dose at 3 AM; for that minority of patients who are unwilling to get up early, the second dose can be taken at 8 AM and the procedures can be scheduled later in the day. The authors recommend the second dose at 3 AM for those whose colonoscopy is scheduled before noon and at 8 AM for those whose procedure is scheduled in the afternoon.

Timing of the split dose and anesthesia
The American Society of Anesthesiologists' guidelines allow, in healthy individuals, the drinking of clear liquids until 2 hours before anesthesia.[25] A split-dose regimen completed 2 hours ahead of the procedure would not interfere with these guidelines. Despite these guidelines, overnight fasting is routinely recommended for patients undergoing colonoscopy with anesthesia because of the fear of aspiration. No difference in the residual gastric volume or gastric pH levels were observed between patients who were allowed to drink clear liquids up to 2 hours before surgery and those who fasted for 6 hours (residual gastric volume: 21 vs 19 mL and pH level: 2.64 vs 2.26).[26] However, patients with delayed emptying of the esophagus or stomach may require longer period of fasting to minimize the risk for aspiration.

Diet on the day before the procedure

Traditionally, patients are instructed to stay on a liquid diet on the day before the colonoscopy. Split dose of PEG-ESL with minimal diet restriction on the day before the procedure have been shown to be effective in cleansing the colon.[20] Recent studies suggest that a low residual diet for breakfast, lunch, and dinner on the day before the procedure and consumption of 4 L of PEG-ESL is comparable to a liquid-diet protocol for colonoscopy preparation.[27]

Simethicone to clear the bubbles

Addition of simethicone to the bowel preparation helps to clear the bubbles and allows better visualization of the colonic mucosa for detection of subtle lesions.[28–31]

Stimulant laxatives as an adjunct

Addition of bisacodyl or extract of *Senna* sp to PEG-ESL helps to clear the stools and improve the quality of colon preparation.[32–35] Use of lubiprostone before split dose of PEG-ESL without dietary restriction has been shown to improve colonic mucosa visualization during colonoscopy.[36] Use of stimulant laxatives as an adjunct to PEG-ESL is helpful in patients with constipation and slow transit.

Timing of colonoscopy after inadequate preparation

About a quarter of the patients with an unacceptable colonic preparation also fail the repeated colonoscopy.[37] Repeating the colonoscopy on the following day immediately after its failure, because of poor preparation, instead of repeating the procedure several weeks later, could reduce the risk for unsatisfactory second preparation.[37]

Customize the preparation

Factors responsible for inadequate colonic preparation include delayed start of colonoscopy, failure to follow preparation instructions, inpatient status, constipation, medications such as tricyclic antidepressants, male gender, and a history of cirrhosis, stroke, dementia, or obesity. In such cases, one may have to customize the protocol of colon preparation by the use of prokinetics to prevent nausea and emesis or by the addition of stimulant or osmotic laxatives to ensure excellent results.[38,39]

Patient education

The importance of colon cleansing for colon cancer prevention and the consequences of suboptimal colonoscopy should be emphasized in patient education. Written material and time for questioning to avoid misunderstanding should be provided. In a prospective study, a patient-education program for endoscopy reduced the rate of failure of procedures caused by poor colon preparation in ambulatory patients from 26% to 4%.[40] The authors show video clips of excellent preparation of the colon along with subtle flat lesions detected during colonoscopy to patients as a part of their counseling about the procedure to improve the patients' compliance with the preparation.

HOW DO WE PREPARE THE PATIENT FOR COLONOSCOPY?

At the authors' institution, the split-dose bowel preparation regimen was implemented in April 2009, based on the preparation developed at the University of Texas Medical Branch (**Fig. 3**). The regimen consists of PEG-ESL solution, bisacodyl tablets, and simethicone. A light breakfast and liquid lunch is recommended on the day before the colonoscopy. In addition, 2 tablets of bisacodyl are given at noon and at 4 PM. The first dose of PEG-ESL (2 L) is given at 4:30 PM. Simethicone is given with the first dose of PEG-ESL. On the day of the procedure, the second dose of PEG is given

COLONOSCOPY PREP MADE EASY
A CLEAN COLON IS CRITICAL FOR COLON CANCER DETECTION

Colon cancer screening involves two steps. The first step is *colon cleansing*, which is critical for the second step that involves *examination of the entire colon*. Unless the colon is absolutely clean, there is no point in going through the procedure.

Follow the steps on the right for colon cleansing

Your bowel movements in the morning after the 2nd dose of GoLYTELY should be *clean*. With *CLEAN PREPARATION* you should be able to see the bottom of the toilet bowl through the liquid as shown below. If it is *NOT CLEAN PREPARATION* you will not be able to see through the liquid.

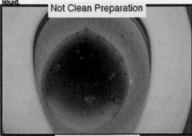
Not Clean Preparation

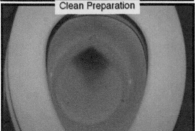
Clean Preparation

If it is *NOT CLEAN PREPARATION* after the second 2 liters of GoLYTELY in the morning, drink another liter of clear fluid or more until it becomes *CLEAR* or *CLEAN PREPARATION* or inform the endoscopy nurse on your arrival to the endoscopy unit.

THE WEEK BEFORE THE PROCEDURE
1. Arrange a driver to bring you to the procedure. The procedure cannot be done without a driver accompanying you.
2. Stop aspirin and iron tablets one week before the procedure. Consult your MD about what to do with holding Coumadin and Plavix and about your diabetes medications.
3. Buy a gallon of GoLYTELY, six tablets of Dulcolax, Gas-X tablets, Vaseline, Tucks medicated pads, Depends diapers.

THE DAY BEFORE THE PROCEDURE - AM
1. Breakfast - Eat light. You can have cereal (without nuts) and milk. You can have orange juice without pulp, coffee, or tea.

THE DAY BEFORE THE PROCEDURE - Noon
1. Lunch - Eat light. You are permitted to have any soup with no vegetables. You are allowed tea or soda.
2. Take two tablets of Dulcolax after lunch.
3. Drink two large glasses of clear liquids (water, ice tea, soda, or gingerale depending on your preference).

THE DAY BEFORE THE PROCEDURE - Evening
1. No dinner.
2. 4:00 PM: Prepare the 4 liters of GoLYTELY solution and keep it in the refrigerator.
3. 4.30 PM: Take two tablets of Dulcolax.
4. 5.00 PM: Drink two liters of GoLYTELY over a couple of hours and keep the rest for AM dose. Also chew a Gas-X tablet.

THE NIGHT BEFORE THE PROCEDURE
Tips to prevent irritation to the anal area
1. Apply vaseline to the anal area and its surrounding area before the first bowel movement to prevent irritation.
2. Use Tucks or a wet soft cloth to gently clean the anal area after bowel movements. Avoid tissue because it can irritate the skin after repeated use.
3. Wear Depends at night to avoid accidental soiling of the bed.

ON THE DAY OF THE PROCEDURE
If your procedure is scheduled before 12 noon.
3:00 AM to 4:00 AM: Take two tablets of Dulcolax and drink the remaining 2 liters of GoLYTELY in 2 hours.
If your procedure is scheduled after 12 noon.
8:00 to 9:00 AM: Take two tablets of Dulcolax and drink the remaining 2 liters of GoLYTELY in 2 hours.
Chew a Gas-X tablet.
You may consider wearing Depends to avoid an accident with your bowel movements on the way to the procedure.
You may take your morning BP and heart medications.

Fig. 3. Split-dose GoLYTELY (Braintree Laboratories Inc) preparation. (*Courtesy of* University of Texas Medical Branch at Galveston; with permission.)

between 3 and 4 AM for those whose colonoscopy is scheduled in the morning, or between 8 and 9 AM for those whose procedure is scheduled in the afternoon.

HOW DO WE EXAMINE THE COLON?
Colonoscopic-Examination Technique

The authors' protocol for colonoscopy is summarized.

1. Colonoscope insertion: A pediatric colonoscope is routinely used for screening the colon. The patient is positioned in the left lateral position. Several measures are undertaken, in addition to the insertion of the endoscope in the cecum, to clear the colon of all the fluid and bubbles for an excellent examination of the colon wall for flat lesions on withdrawal (**Fig. 4**).

2. Suction and clearance of fluid during endoscope insertion: Instead of attempting to reach the cecum as fast as possible, time is taken to wash and suction the residual fluid completely on the way to the cecum. A clean colon helps in the use of additional techniques such as electronic or dye-stained chromoendoscopy (**Fig. 5**).

3. Simethicone flush to clear the bubbles: Another technique routinely used is the flushing of simethicone (30 ml of Simethicone flush [30 ml of water mixed with a few drops of Simethicone solution]) in the sigmoid colon, proximal transverse colon, and cecum and ascending colon to clear the bubbles in the colon. Flushing is done as the endoscope is inserted into the cecum, so that during the withdrawal the colonic mucosa is clear and free from bubbles (**Fig. 6**).

4. Working the folds: Because the angle of view of the colonoscope is less than 180°, simply withdrawing the colonoscope in the center of the lumen will miss colonic lesions. Instead, one should work the folds and make an attempt to examine carefully the interhaustral areas.

5. To-and-fro movement: In addition to working the folds, it is critical to gently move the scope to-and-fro using gentle intermittent suction, if necessary, to appreciate the subtle mucosal changes of flat lesions. Also, as one comes down a bend, the outer wall is seen easily. The blind spots should be examined by pushing the endoscope in again.

6. Limiting colonic contractions by avoiding vigorous suction during endoscope withdrawal: By clearing all the fluid and bubbles during the colonoscope insertion and having a relatively dry and clear field ready for examination during the

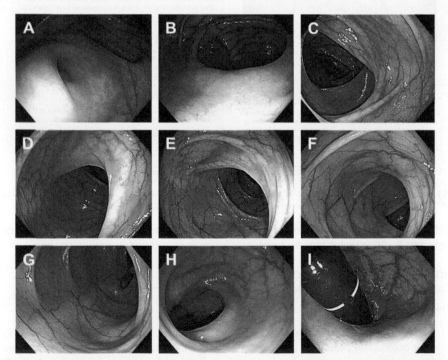

Fig. 4. (*A–I*) BBPS score of 3 out of 3 in the right, transverse, and left colon. Careful examination of the colon wall is possible for flat lesions in addition to the lumen for polypoid lesions.

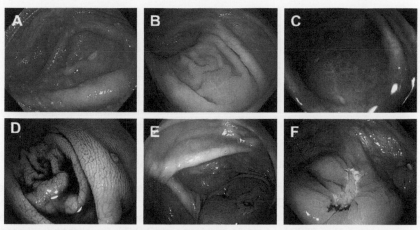

Fig. 5. The importance of clean bowel preparation. Excellent bowel preparation is critical to the detection of NP-CRN. The flat adenoma would have been missed if the cecum (*A*) had not been properly washed and suctioned (*B*). The stool would have obscured visualization and examination of the lesion using narrow-band imaging (*C*) because bile and stool appear reddish under narrow-band imaging. The stool would also hinder the application of diluted indigo carmine (*D*) and make endoscopic resection more challenging (*E, F*). (*Courtesy of* Roy Soetikno, MD, Palo Alto Veteran's Hospital, Palo Alto.)

endoscope withdrawal, there would be no or minimal need for suction and a relatively stable field for examination without any interference from vigorous peristalsis.

7. Position change: Changing the position of the patient to supine and right lateral as the endoscope is withdrawn to the left colon, allows the left colon to remain distended (the left colon, being nondependent, distends better in the right lateral position than in the left lateral position), thus making a larger surface area of the colon available for screening.

8. Focus on the vascular network: Unlike the pedunculated and sessile polyps, which are easily visible during endoscopy, detection of the flat lesions requires a focused examination of the vascular network for subtle changes or loss of vascular network under the flat lesion (**Fig. 7**).

9. Strolling back slowly: Strolling back slowly with the endoscope is critical for screening as there is a lot of surface area to be screened.

10. Training nurses and technicians to detect flat lesions: Despite the best efforts of the endoscopists, they can lose focus transiently and miss lesions. The rate of NP-CRN detection increases with the active participation, during the colonoscopy, of nurses and technicians who are trained in the detection of these lesions.

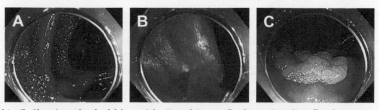

Fig. 6. (*A–C*) Clearing the bubbles with simethicone flush to visualize flat lesions.

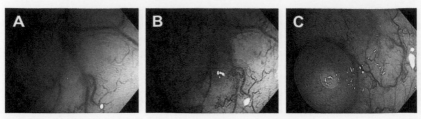

Fig. 7. Subtle lesion overlying and obscuring the blood vessels.

BETTER PREPARATION, BETTER EXAMINATION, BETTER ADENOMA DETECTION

An observation study of patients undergoing screening colonoscopies at the University of Texas M.D. Anderson Cancer Center using the colon preparation and colonoscopic screening technique described in the previous section was carried out from February to November 2009 by a single endoscopist (G.S.R.). Excellent bowel preparation (BBPS score of 7–9) was achieved in 167 of 170 (98%) patients. The median insertion time was 11 minutes (range 2–45 minutes) and total procedure time was 39 minutes (range 17–90 minutes). The adenoma detection rate was 50 of 77 (65%) in men and 45 of 93 (48%) in women. Of the 356 polyps detected, 13 were pedunculated polyps, 120 were flat lesions, and 223 were sessile polyps. Ninety-two patients (54%) had 1 flat lesion detected during colonoscopy.[41]

SUMMARY

A clean, dry colon is critical for the detection of non-polypoid lesions and can be achieved with a split dose of PEG-ESL in most patients. In addition, the endoscopist should use simethicone to clear the bubbles, should suction any residual fluid during colonoscope insertion, and should screen carefully, working the folds to detect flat lesions.

REFERENCES

1. Robertson DJ, Greenberg ER, Beach M, et al. Colorectal cancer in patients under close colonoscopic surveillance. Gastroenterology 2005;129(1):34–41.
2. Lieberman D. A call to action—measuring the quality of colonoscopy. N Engl J Med 2006;355(24):2588–9.
3. Jass JR. Colorectal cancer: a multipathway disease. Crit Rev Oncog 2006; 12(3–4):273–87.
4. Kudo S, Lambert R, Allen JI, et al. Nonpolypoid neoplastic lesions of the colorectal mucosa. Gastrointest Endosc 2008;68(Suppl 4):S3–47.
5. Endoscopic Classification Review Group. Update on the Paris classification of superficial neoplastic lesions in the digestive tract. Endoscopy 2005;37(6):570–8.
6. Soetikno RM, Kaltenbach T, Rouse RV, et al. Prevalence of nonpolypoid (flat and depressed) colorectal neoplasms in asymptomatic and symptomatic adults. JAMA 2008;299(9):1027–35.
7. Burke CA, Church JM. Enhancing the quality of colonoscopy: the importance of bowel purgatives. Gastrointest Endosc 2007;66(3):565–73.
8. Harewood GC, Sharma VK, de Garmo P. Impact of colonoscopy preparation quality on detection of suspected colonic neoplasia. Gastrointest Endosc 2003; 58(1):76–9.
9. Froehlich F, Wietlisbach V, Gonvers JJ, et al. Impact of colonic cleansing on quality and diagnostic yield of colonoscopy: the European Panel of Appropriateness of

Gastrointestinal Endoscopy European multicenter study. Gastrointest Endosc 2005;61(3):378–84.

10. Rex DK. Maximizing detection of adenomas and cancers during colonoscopy. Am J Gastroenterol 2006;101(12):2866–77.

11. Parra-Blanco A, Nicolas-Perez D, Gimeno-Garcia A, et al. The timing of bowel preparation before colonoscopy determines the quality of cleansing, and is a significant factor contributing to the detection of flat lesions: a randomized study. World J Gastroenterol 2006;12(38):6161–6.

12. Winawer SJ, Zauber AG, Fletcher RH, et al. Guidelines for colonoscopy surveillance after polypectomy: a consensus update by the US Multi-Society Task Force on Colorectal Cancer and the American Cancer Society. Gastroenterology 2006; 130(6):1872–85.

13. Alert F. Oral sodium phosphate (OSP) products for bowel cleansing. 2008. Available at: http://www.fda.gov/cder/drug/infopage/OSP_solution/default.htm. Accessed May 17, 2009.

14. Hayes A, Buffum M, Fuller D. Bowel preparation comparison: flavored versus unflavored colyte. Gastroenterol Nurs 2003;26(3):106–9.

15. Matter SE, Rice PS, Campbell DR. Colonic lavage solutions: plain versus flavored. Am J Gastroenterol 1993;88(1):49–52.

16. Rostom A, Jolicoeur E. Validation of a new scale for the assessment of bowel preparation quality. Gastrointest Endosc 2004;59(4):482–6.

17. Lai EJ, Calderwood AH, Doros G, et al. The Boston bowel preparation scale: a valid and reliable instrument for colonoscopy-oriented research. Gastrointest Endosc 2009;69(Suppl 3):620–5.

18. Church JM. Effectiveness of polyethylene glycol antegrade gut lavage bowel preparation for colonoscopy—timing is the key! Dis Colon Rectum 1998;41(10): 1223–5.

19. Park JS, Sohn CI, Hwang SJ, et al. Quality and effect of single dose versus split dose of polyethylene glycol bowel preparation for early-morning colonoscopy. Endoscopy 2007;39(7):616–9.

20. El Sayed AM, Kanafani ZA, Mourad FH, et al. A randomized single-blind trial of whole versus split-dose polyethylene glycol-electrolyte solution for colonoscopy preparation. Gastrointest Endosc 2003;58(1):36–40.

21. Di Palma JA, Rodriguez R, McGowan J, et al. A randomized clinical study evaluating the safety and efficacy of a new, reduced-volume, oral sulfate colon-cleansing preparation for colonoscopy. Am J Gastroenterol 2009;104(9): 2275–84.

22. Frommer D. Cleansing ability and tolerance of three bowel preparations for colonoscopy. Dis Colon Rectum 1997;40(1):100–4.

23. Gupta T, Mandot A, Desai D, et al. Comparison of two schedules (previous evening versus same morning) of bowel preparation for colonoscopy. Endoscopy 2007;39(8):706–9.

24. Siddiqui AA, Yang K, Spechler SJ, et al. Duration of the interval between the completion of bowel preparation and the start of colonoscopy predicts bowel-preparation quality. Gastrointest Endosc 2009;69(Suppl 3):700–6.

25. Practice guidelines for preoperative fasting and the use of pharmacologic agents to reduce the risk of pulmonary aspiration: application to healthy patients undergoing elective procedures: a report by the American Society of Anesthesiologist Task Force on Preoperative Fasting. Anesthesiology 1999;90(3):896–905.

26. Phillips S, Hutchinson S, Davidson T. Preoperative drinking does not affect gastric contents. Br J Anaesth 1993;70(1):6–9.

27. Park DI, Park SH, Lee SK, et al. Efficacy of prepackaged, low residual test meals with 4L polyethylene glycol versus a clear liquid diet with 4L polyethylene glycol bowel preparation: a randomized trial. J Gastroenterol Hepatol 2009;24(6): 988–91.

28. Kark W, Krebs-Richter H, Hotz J. [Improving the effect of orthograde colonic lavage with golytely solution by adding dimethicone]. Z Gastroenterol 1995; 33(1):20–3 [in German].

29. Lazzaroni M, Petrillo M, Desideri S, et al. Efficacy and tolerability of polyethylene glycol-electrolyte lavage solution with and without simethicone in the preparation of patients with inflammatory bowel disease for colonoscopy. Aliment Pharmacol Ther 1993;7(6):655–9.

30. Sudduth RH, DeAngelis S, Sherman KE, et al. The effectiveness of simethicone in improving visibility during colonoscopy when given with a sodium phosphate solution: a double-blind randomized study. Gastrointest Endosc 1995;42(5): 413–5.

31. Tongprasert S, Sobhonslidsuk A, Rattanasiri S. Improving quality of colonoscopy by adding simethicone to sodium phosphate bowel preparation. World J Gastroenterol 2009;15(24):3032–7.

32. Clarkston WK, Smith OJ. The use of GoLYTELY and Dulcolax in combination in outpatient colonoscopy. J Clin Gastroenterol 1993;17(2):146–8.

33. Ziegenhagen DJ, Zehnter E, Tacke W, et al. Addition of senna improves colonoscopy preparation with lavage: a prospective randomized trial. Gastrointest Endosc 1991;37(5):547–9.

34. DiPalma JA, McGowan J, Cleveland MV. Clinical trial: an efficacy evaluation of reduced bisacodyl given as part of a polyethylene glycol electrolyte solution preparation prior to colonoscopy. Aliment Pharmacol Ther 2007;26(8):1113–9.

35. DiPalma JA, Wolff BG, Meagher A, et al. Comparison of reduced volume versus four liters sulfate-free electrolyte lavage solutions for colonoscopy colon cleansing. Am J Gastroenterol 2003;98(10):2187–91.

36. Stengel JZ, Jones DP. Single-dose lubiprostone along with split-dose PEG solution without dietary restrictions for bowel cleansing prior to colonoscopy: a randomized, double-blind, placebo-controlled trial. Am J Gastroenterol 2008; 103(9):2224–30.

37. Ben-Horin S, Bar-Meir S, Avidan B. The outcome of a second preparation for colonoscopy after preparation failure in the first procedure. Gastrointest Endosc 2009;69(Suppl 3):626–30.

38. Ness RM, Manam R, Hoen H, et al. Predictors of inadequate bowel preparation for colonoscopy. Am J Gastroenterol 2001;96(6):1797–802.

39. Borg BB, Gupta NK, Zuckerman GR, et al. Impact of obesity on bowel preparation for colonoscopy. Clin Gastroenterol Hepatol 2009;7(6):670–5.

40. Abuksis G, Mor M, Segal N, et al. A patient education program is cost-effective for preventing failure of endoscopic procedures in a gastroenterology department. Am J Gastroenterol 2001;96(6):1786–90.

41. Raju GS, Dasari C, Singh H. Better preparation, better screening, better adenoma detection. Gastrointest Endosc 2010;71:AB328.

Development of Expertise in the Detection and Classification of Non-Polypoid Colorectal Neoplasia: Experience-Based Data at an Academic GI Unit

Silvia Sanduleanu, MD, PhD*, Eveline J.A. Rondagh, MD,
Ad. A.M. Masclee, MD, PhD

KEYWORDS

- Colorectal cancer • Colorectal adenomas
- Non-polypoid colorectal neoplasia
- Flat adenomas • GI training

Colorectal cancer (CRC) is an important health care issue worldwide.[1] According to the World Health Organization, there are approximately 1,000,000 new diagnoses of CRC each year, with mortality of more than 500,000.[2] The socioeconomic impact of this problem provided the drive for rapidly expanding screening programs. In general, accurate detection and removal of the precursor lesions—colorectal adenomas—are considered to be powerful tools for fighting against CRC.[3] Unexpectedly, however, in routine practice, the protection against CRC offered by colonoscopic screening is far from perfect.[4–7] A recent study by Baxter and colleagues[7] demonstrated that although colonoscopy was associated with decreased risk of subsequent CRC in the distal colon, no protective effect was found against cancers located on the right side of the colon. Why may colonoscopy so far fail to prevent CRCs?

Department of Internal Medicine, Division of Gastroenterology and Hepatology, Maastricht University Medical Center, PO Box 5800, 6202 AZ Maastricht, The Netherlands
* Corresponding author.
E-mail address: s.sanduleanu@mumc.nl

Gastrointest Endoscopy Clin N Am 20 (2010) 449–460
doi:10.1016/j.giec.2010.03.006
1052-5157/10/$ – see front matter © 2010 Elsevier Inc. All rights reserved.

Some polyps are simply not recognized because of patient-related factors, eg, suboptimal bowel preparation, inefficient withdrawal technique, or difficult anatomic conditions.[8,9] Other polyps are missed as a consequence of insufficient awareness and training of the endoscopist, non-polypoid colorectal neoplasms (NP-CRNs) being an illustrative example in this regard.[10,11] An increasing body of evidence presently indicates that NP-CRNs are common lesions worldwide.[12–25] Detection and management of some of these lesions may prove to be more challenging, raising the hypothesis that these lesions may be at the origin of interval cancers.

In addition, surveillance practices after polypectomy are based on clinicopathologic features of adenomas, namely size, multiplicity, presence of any villous component, and grade of dysplasia.[3,26] Unfortunately, evaluation and recording of these features in routine practice frequently lack precision and proper standardization, making it difficult to draw firm conclusions regarding follow-up intervals. All of these practical limitations eventually highlight the need to secure the quality of colonoscopic examination if interval cancers are to be prevented. It is reasonable to presume that high-quality colonoscopic practices will offer in turn considerable potential to refine the diagnosis of colorectal neoplasia, and, hence, to delineate subgroups of patients truly at risk for developing CRC. Implementation of such risk-stratification strategies and personalized medical care can ultimately lead to appropriate redirection of the limited economic resources.[26]

At its core, quality improvement in gastrointestinal (GI) practice relies on continuous training, education, and information among all health care providers, whether gastroenterologists, GI trainees, endoscopy nurses, or GI pathologists. Over the past few years, it became clear that objective criteria are needed to assess the quality of colonoscopy, such as cecum intubation rate, quality of bowel preparation, withdrawal time, and adenoma detection rate.[8] In this context, development of competence among practicing endoscopists to adequately detect and treat NP-CRNs deserves special attention. We describe a summary of the path to develop expertise in detection and management of NP-CRNs, based on experience at our academic GI unit.

THE LEARNING PYRAMID

For simplicity, let's look at the well-known learning-pyramid by Miller,[27] as illustrated in **Fig. 1**. In general, development of practical skills is a stepwise process, starting with acquisition of *basic knowledge*, followed by in-depth information and development of practical skills—the so-called *know-how* and *show-how*—and finally exposure to concrete practical situations. If we extrapolate this model to the practice of GI endoscopy, in particular development of expertise in diagnosis of NP-CRN, the following scenarios are possible:

- Imagine you are supervising a young GI trainee who performs a colonoscopy. The trainee tells you he or she identified a lesion in the right colon, but cannot find it again during withdrawal. You take over, but also without success. Three years later the patient is diagnosed with an interval cancer, probably emerging from a missed lesion at the same location. What would you do now? You would probably seek to review literature data pertaining to origins of interval cancers and discuss these with your students to improve clinical awareness in this regard.
- Imagine again you are supervising a more experienced trainee. The trainee detects a large lesion with apparently flat morphology, but unfortunately he or she is not able to find it again during withdrawal. You tell the trainee that some

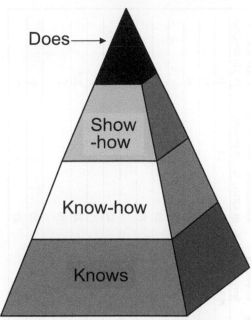

Fig. 1. Learning pyramid by Miller. (*Adapted from* Miller AG. The assessment of clinical skills/competence/performance. Acad Med 1990;65:S63–7; with permission.)

of these lesions may herald the risk to more rapidly evolve into CRC. You take over and after careful inspection and selective chromoendoscopy, find a lateral spreading polyp, and remove it. It turns out to be a high-grade dysplastic adenoma. It is clear that mastering know-how about detection and showing how these lesions should be correctly managed are essential steps in providing endoscopy training in this regard.

- Now imagine that the same trainee (meanwhile in the past year) detects a lesion and after evaluation with selective chromoendoscopy, describes it as a flat lesion with a central depression. The trainee properly lifts it with NaCl 9% and removes it in toto. It turns out to be a high-grade dysplastic adenoma. You tell the trainee that he or she did a very good job!

THE DEVELOPMENT OF THE DE NOVO EXPERTISE IN NP-CRN AT MAASTRICHT

In real life, the issue of developing expertise in detection and management of NP-CRN in current practice can be broken down into a number of questions.

Why is Knowledge About NP-CRN Important?

Without a proper understanding of the clinical relevance of NP-CRNs, it is impossible to say whether concerns related to underdetection of these lesions are legitimate or whether these reflect semantic differences only. The earliest reports concerning NP-CRNs coincided with technological progress in GI endoscopy, namely use of chromoendoscopy, magnification techniques, and high-resolution imaging.[13,28–30] Numerous studies dating back to the early 1990s correlated some of these lesions with more aggressive histopathological features.[12,31] **Table 1** provides an overview of some of these studies, with focus on methodology, prevalence of CRNs in general,

Table 1
Overview of clinical studies addressing prevalence of NP-CRNs worldwide

Author, Country, Publication	No. of Patients	Mean Age, y	Gender, % Males	Indication Symptoms, %	Screening Surveillance, %	Total Prevalence of CRNs, %	Prevalence of NP-CRNs, %	Prevalence of HGD/Early CRC (%) in NP-CRNs
Jaramillo et al[13] (UK), Gastrointest Endosc 1995[a]	232	62	43	67	30	41	24	14
Fujii et al[14] (UK), Endoscopy 1998[a]	208	58	41	43	48[b]	22	-	11
Rembacken et al[15] (UK), Lancet 2000[a]	1000	59	41	69	27[b]	23	-	16
Saitoh et al[16] (USA), Gastroenterology 2001	211	58	36	57	33	38	-	-
Tsuda et al[17] (Sweden), Gut 2002[a]	866	67[c]	51[c]	57[c]	38[c]	39	6	24
Hurlstone et al[18] (UK), Am J Gastroenterol 2003[a]	850	60	53	43	53	70	-	27
Diebold et al[19] (Fr), Am J Gastroenterol 2004[a]	133[c]	62[c]	71[c]	45[c]	42[c]	-	-	18
Soetikno et al[20] (USA), JAMA 2008[a]	1819	64	95	30	70	42	9	7
Park et al[21] (S-Korea), Dis Colon Rectum 2008	3360[c]	57[c]	71[c]	31[c]	45[c]	-	-	5[d]
Kil Lee et al[22] (Korea), Scand J Gastroenterol 2008	8593	59[c]	70[c]	-	>25[c]	27	3[d]	20[d]
Chiu et al[23] (China), Clin Gastroenterol Hepatol 2009[a]	12,731	51	56	0	100	19	4	3
Kim et al[24] (USA), Colorectal Dis 2009[a]	642	59	43	-	100	20	6	0
Rondagh et al[25] (NL), 2009, submitted[a]	2310	58	46	79	21	27	4	16

Abbreviations: CRC, colorectal cancer; HGD, high-grade dysplasia; NP-CRNs, non-polypoid colorectal neoplasms.
[a] Mean prevalence of HGD/early CRC in Paris type II-c lesions found in these studies was 55% (ranges, 0%–100%).
[b] Including ulcerative colitis surveillance.
[c] Demographic data from patients with adenomas.
[d] Only lesions ≥5 mm included.

prevalence of NP-CRNs, and association with severe histopathology. Pooling data from these studies, it appears that prevalence of NP-CRNs ranges from 3% to 24% (mean, 8.1%), while prevalence of Paris type II-c lesions is very low (1%–2%);[32] however, a large proportion of Paris type II-c lesions harbor advanced histopathology (mean prevalence, 55.4%, range 0%–100%). The clinical message emerging from these studies is that (1) *prevalence* of NP-CRNs in the Western population is *comparable* with the initially reported data from Japan: the relatively wide variation in prevalence among different studies may reflect dissent in endoscopic definition and geographic differences, but most probably different levels of clinical awareness, education, and training; (2) a subset of these lesions is more difficult to *detect* and to *manage* endoscopically; (3) also, a subset of these lesions, especially Paris type II-c, although relatively uncommon, are more frequently associated with *advanced histopathology*. Given the expected increase in incidence of CRC in the foreseeable future, and the major impact of colonoscopic screening on GI practices worldwide, it is mandatory to provide our trainees with appropriate education in this regard.

How Can We Develop Expertise in Detection of Flat Adenomas?

Traditionally, education and training in GI endoscopy were practice-based. Nowadays, the theory and practice of education are undergoing fundamental changes. Multimedia information systems are facilitating continuous updating and pooling of information and knowledge. The expansion of teleteaching, telelearning, and teleconferencing over the past years permits virtual connection and *real-time* dialog of gastroenterologists, worldwide.[33,34] This allows transfer of knowledge and experience from expertise centers to academic or nonacademic GI practices, without limits of distance or borders. In an original study, Kaltenbach and colleagues[35] addressed the role of teleteaching in GI endoscopy. Live, interactive, high-resolution, uncompressed video transmission was used, by means of digital video transport systems. Trainees, faculty, and staff at 3 international endoscopy units participated in this prospective study. Prelecture and postlecture scores were recorded, showing that this model is technically feasible and highly efficient in GI endoscopy training, at affordable costs. Alternatively, simulator training has evolved over the past years faster than before.[36] A Dutch study using the Symbionix GI Mentor II simulator (Simbionix Ltd, Israel) advocates implementation of this program in training of novice endoscopists.[37] Further development of this software may also help endoscopists achieve competence regarding recognition and treatment of NP-CRNs. Conceivably, testing and continuous evaluation of knowledge and practical skills in this field are essential to maintain adequate educational level.

In an attempt to improve the quality of colonoscopic examination, with emphasis on detection of NP-CRNs, we have undertaken a prospective study at our academic center. **Fig. 2** depicts the study design. Before beginning this study, a series of topic lectures were presented by a dedicated colonoscopist (S.S.) to provide general theoretical insight into the epidemiology and pathophysiology, including molecular aspects, clinical detection, and endoscopic removal of these lesions. Video training was then offered using accredited programs,[38,39] as well as continuous feedback and supervision during endoscopy. Finally, all 16 endoscopists at our GI unit, 9 staff members and 7 trainees, embarked on this study, addressing the prevalence and clinicopathologic features of NP-CRNs in a Dutch population. Between February 2008 and February 2009, clinical, endoscopic, and histopathological data from 2310 consecutive patients referred for routine colonoscopy were recorded. Standardized endoscopy reports, including digital photographic documentation, were available from all patients. Special attention was paid to recording of quality indicators. Our

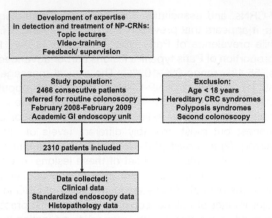

Fig. 2. Algorithm of study design.

GI endoscopy unit offers secondary and tertiary care, and serves a total population of approximately 200,000. To ensure accurate classification of flat lesions in this nonexpert setting, a simplified definition was used, as previously proposed.[11] **Table 2** summarizes the characteristics of the study population.

What Do We Have to Know About Treatment of These Lesions?

Literature data are available in this regard,[40,41] (see the articles by Kaltenbach and Soetikno; and Saito and colleagues elsewhere in this issue for further exploration of this topic). Before beginning our study, we reviewed basic principles regarding detection, classification, and management of non-polypoid lesions. In addition, using video training programs, we learned some practical tips regarding detection of NP-CRNs. Besides careful inspection, dynamic evaluation of focal lesions after insufflation/desufflation of air can assist in evaluation of morphology, and eventually allow visualization of a central depression. Selective chromoendoscopy using indigo-carmine 0.4% was used to better delineate the borders before endoscopic removal (**Fig. 3**). To reduce peristalsis, enhance visualization of lesions, and facilitate their removal, buthylscopolamine was injected intravenously, when indicated. The authors used the inject-and-cut endoscopic mucosal resection (EMR) technique to resect NP-CRNs, as described elsewhere.[42] Lesions that could not be managed

Table 2	
Characteristics of study population	
No. of patients	2310
Males (%)	46.1
Age, y, mean (range)	58.4 (18–93)
Indication colonoscopy	
• Symptoms, %	79.4
• Screening/surveillance, %	20.6
Previous history of CRC, %	3.1
Familial CRC, %	1.9
Inflammatory bowel diseases, %	9.8
Patients with ≥1 adenoma, %	26.8
Patients with ≥1 flat adenoma, %	4.2

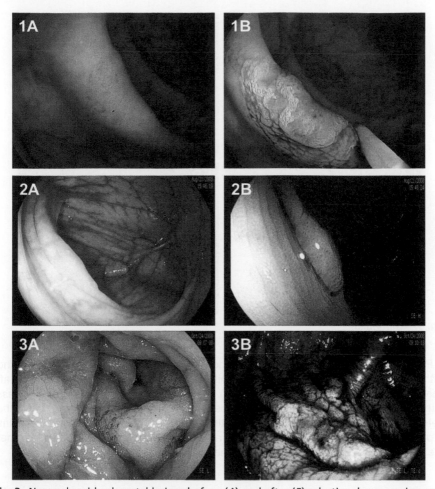

Fig. 3. Non-polypoid colorectal lesions before (*A*) and after (*B*) selective chromoendoscopy. (*1*) Non-polypoid Paris type 0-IIa colorectal lesion found in the ascending colon. Selective chromoendoscopy clarified the borders of the lesion, thereby facilitating the removal. Histological examination showed a tubular adenoma with low-grade dysplasia. (*2*) Non-polypoid lesion detected at the hepatic flexure after applying selective chromoendoscopy. Histological examination showed a hyperplastic polyp. (*3*) Lateral spreading tumor of granular type detected in the cecum. Histological examination of the surgical specimen showed a tubulo-villous adenoma with high-grade dysplasia. (*4*) Large non-polypoid lesion in the ascending colon with mucus layer on top of lesion, suggesting a sessile serrated adenoma. (*5*) Diminutive non-polypoid lesion detected in the ascending colon. Histological examination showed a tubular adenoma with low-grade dysplasia.

endoscopically were marked with ink to assist the surgeon during subsequent intraoperative removal.

What Is the Learning Curve for the Endoscopist?

So far, studies that systematically address this issue have not been published. Nevertheless, given rapidly growing literature data within this field, this question should be relatively easy and inexpensive to answer.

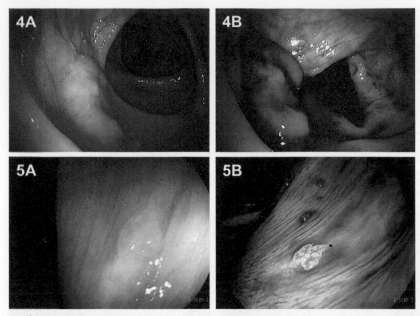

Fig. 3. (*continued*)

Perhaps not surprisingly, in our experience, after relatively short, intensive training with regard to recognition of NP-CRNs, similar detection rates were found among staff gastroenterologists and GI trainees (**Fig. 4**). Hence, it appears that *clinical awareness* rather than *general experience* of the endoscopist is likely to play a critical role in the detection of these lesions. Another interesting aspect is that prevalence of flat lesions in our study population (4.2%) was comparable with prevalence data reported in other Western populations, further supporting the efficacy of this training model.

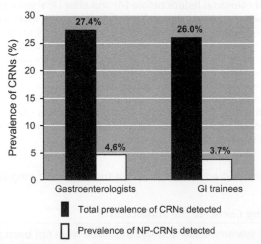

Fig. 4. Similar detection rates of total CRNs and of NP-CRNs were found among staff gastroenterologists and GI trainees.

Should Detection of Flat Adenomas Be a Quality Indicator in Training of GI Endoscopists?

Probably yes, albeit the expected prevalence may be subject to large variation and remains to be further defined. Reporting of prevalence of flat adenomas should be probably related to other quality indicators. In our experience, the cecum intubation rate was 90.2% in the symptomatic population, and 95.0% in the screening/surveillance population, which is in agreement with international recommendations. Also, we reported an adenoma prevalence of 33.7% in males and of 20.9% in females older than 50 years, which is higher than the reported average data.[9]

What Are Some of the Unanswered Questions About NP-CRN Today?

First, the question arises whether morphologic classification of colorectal lesions, according to the Paris classification, should be regarded as a valuable clinical instrument or rather a scientific one. As this classification is based on expert opinions, its prospective validation is needed in the future. One may argue that proper classification of colorectal lesions is likely to increase precision and uniformity in recording of data, and hence may allow fine tuning of surveillance programs. In view of this, it is probably also an important step in education of GI trainees. A second question is whether flat or sessile morphology makes any difference in small lesions. Because there is relatively much room for subjective interpretation in this regard, it is reasonable to assume that such differentiation is less important when it concerns Paris type II-a (flat, elevated) lesions. Efforts should be made, however, to detect, accurately classify, and completely remove even small type II-b or II-c lesions, as these are associated with more severe histopathology. Third, it would be desirable to define in the future risk groups that are more likely to herald non-polypoid colorectal lesions. Special attention should be offered to patients with hereditary forms of CRC, in particular those with Lynch syndrome, as they seem to frequently harbor such lesions.[43,44] Associations of NP-CRNs with different phenotypic or genotypic features may permit customizing of screening recommendations, and, hence, increase the efficiency of screening programs. Finally, prospective, follow-up studies of patients harboring NP-CRNs are needed to bring more light on the biologic behavior of these lesions. Needless to say, all these issues can be clarified only if gastroenterologists and pathologists will join in their efforts to diagnose and classify colorectal neoplasia as objectively, uniformly, and reliably as possible.

SUMMARY

Based on sound clinical data, we can conclude that accurate detection of NP-CRNs is important and should be incorporated into GI educational programs. Diagnosis and management of some of these lesions in routine practice may be technically challenging. Also, a subset of these lesions may herald advanced histopathology. Our experience in this field adds a further piece of evidence to the mosaic of clinical data indicating that worldwide training in recognition and management of NP-CRNs warrants further consideration if prevention of CRC is to be optimized. It is plausible that *clinical awareness* prevails upon *experience* in diagnosis of these lesions, although this hypothesis should be further tested. Finally, the key message for the endoscopist, irrespective of level of education and practical experience, is that continuously training and "retraining our eyes" is important not only for saving more lives, but also for learning new essential lessons about CRC prevention.

REFERENCES

1. Jemal A, Siegel R, Ward E, et al. Cancer statistics, 2009. CA Cancer J Clin 2009; 59:225–49.
2. Ferlay J, Bray F, Pisani P, et al. GLOBOCAN 2002: Cancer incidence, mortality and prevalence worldwide. Lyon (France): IARCPress; 2004. IARC CancerBase No. 5. version 2.0.
3. Winawer SJ, Zauber AG, Ho MN, et al. Prevention of colorectal cancer by colonoscopic polypectomy. The National Polyp Study Workgroup. N Engl J Med 1993; 329:1977–81.
4. Singh H, Turner D, Xue L, et al. Risk of developing colorectal cancer following a negative colonoscopy examination: evidence for a 10-year interval between colonoscopies. JAMA 2006;295:2366–73.
5. Bressler B, Paszat LF, Chen Z, et al. Rates of new or missed colorectal cancers after colonoscopy and their risk factors: a population-based analysis. Gastroenterology 2007;132:96–102.
6. Lakoff J, Paszat LF, Saskin R, et al. Risk of developing proximal versus distal colorectal cancer after a negative colonoscopy: a population-based study. Clin Gastroenterol Hepatol 2008;6:1117–21.
7. Baxter NN, Goldwasser MA, Paszat LF, et al. Association of colonoscopy and death from colorectal cancer. Ann Intern Med 2009;150:1–8.
8. Rex DK, Cutler CS, Lemmel GT, et al. Colonoscopic miss rates of adenomas determined by back-to-back colonoscopies. Gastroenterology 1997;112:24–8.
9. Rex DK, Petrini JL, Baron TH, et al. Quality indicators for colonoscopy. Gastrointest Endosc 2006;63:S16–28.
10. Kudo S, Lambert R, Allen JI, et al. Nonpolypoid neoplastic lesions of the colorectal mucosa. Gastrointest Endosc 2008;68:S3–47.
11. Soetikno R, Friedland S, Kaltenbach T, et al. Nonpolypoid (flat and depressed) colorectal neoplasms. Gastroenterology 2006;130:566–76, quiz 588–9.
12. Kudo S, Kashida H, Tamura T, et al. Colonoscopic diagnosis and management of nonpolypoid early colorectal cancer. World J Surg 2000;24:1081–90.
13. Jaramillo E, Watanabe M, Slezak P, et al. Flat neoplastic lesions of the colon and rectum detected by high-resolution video endoscopy and chromoscopy. Gastrointest Endosc 1995;42:114–22.
14. Fujii T, Rembacken BJ, Dixon MF, et al. Flat adenomas in the United Kingdom: are treatable cancers being missed? Endoscopy 1998;30:437–43.
15. Rembacken BJ, Fujii T, Cairns A, et al. Flat and depressed colonic neoplasms: a prospective study of 1000 colonoscopies in the UK. Lancet 2000;355: 1211–4.
16. Saitoh Y, Waxman I, West AB, et al. Prevalence and distinctive biologic features of flat colorectal adenomas in a North American population. Gastroenterology 2001; 120:1657–65.
17. Tsuda S, Veress B, Toth E, et al. Flat and depressed colorectal tumours in a southern Swedish population: a prospective chromoendoscopic and histopathological study. Gut 2002;51:550–5.
18. Hurlstone DP, Cross SS, Adam I, et al. A prospective clinicopathological and endoscopic evaluation of flat and depressed colorectal lesions in the United Kingdom. Am J Gastroenterol 2003;98:2543–9.
19. Diebold MD, Samalin E, Merle C, et al. Flat neoplasia: frequency and concordance between endoscopic appearance and histological diagnosis in a French prospective series. Am J Gastroenterol 2004;99:1795–800.

20. Soetikno RM, Kaltenbach T, Rouse RV, et al. Prevalence of nonpolypoid (flat and depressed) colorectal neoplasms in asymptomatic and symptomatic adults. Jama 2008;299:1027–35.
21. Park DH, Kim HS, Kim WH, et al. Clinicopathologic characteristics and malignant potential of colorectal flat neoplasia compared with that of polypoid neoplasia. Dis Colon Rectum 2008;51:43–9 [discussion: 49].
22. Kil Lee S, Il Kim T, Kwan Shin S, et al. Comparison of the clinicopathologic features between flat and polypoid adenoma. Scand J Gastroenterol 2008;43: 1116–21.
23. Chiu H-M, Lin J-T, Chen C-C, et al. Prevalence and characteristics of nonpolypoid colorectal neoplasm in an asymptomatic and average-risk Chinese population. Clin Gastroenterol Hepatol 2009;7:463–70.
24. Kim J, Rami P, O'Toole J, et al. Prevalence and size of flat neoplasms in a heterogeneous population undergoing routine colorectal cancer screening. Colorectal Dis 2009;2:471–6.
25. Rondagh E, van der Valk M, Winkens B, et al. S. Nonpolypoid (flat and depressed) colorectal neoplasms in women are more likely to contain advanced histology [abstract]. DDW 2010.
26. Winawer S, Fletcher R, Rex D, et al. Colorectal cancer screening and surveillance: clinical guidelines and rationale-update based on new evidence. Gastroenterology 2003;124:544–60.
27. Miller GE. The assessment of clinical skills/competence/performance. Acad Med 1990;65:S63–7.
28. Muto T, Kamiya J, Sawada T, et al. Small "flat adenoma" of the large bowel with special reference to its clinicopathologic features. Dis Colon Rectum 1985;28: 847–51.
29. Kudo S, Tamura S, Hirota S, et al. The problem of de novo colorectal carcinoma. Eur J Cancer 1995;31A:1118–20.
30. Tanaka S, Haruma K, Oka S, et al. Clinicopathologic features and endoscopic treatment of superficially spreading colorectal neoplasms larger than 20 mm. Gastrointest Endosc 2001;54:62–6.
31. Leong AF, Seow-Choen F, Tang CL. Diminutive cancers of the colon and rectum: comparison between flat and polypoid cancers. Int J Colorectal Dis 1998;13:151–3.
32. The Paris endoscopic classification of superficial neoplastic lesions: esophagus, stomach, and colon: November 30 to December 1, 2002. Gastrointest Endosc 2003;58:S3–43.
33. Strode SW, Gustke S, Allen A. Technical and clinical progress in telemedicine. Jama 1999;281:1066–8.
34. Rabenstein T, Maiss J, Naegele-Jackson S, et al. Tele-endoscopy: influence of data compression, bandwidth and simulated impairments on the usability of real-time digital video endoscopy transmissions for medical diagnoses. Endoscopy 2002;34:703–10.
35. Kaltenbach T, Muto M, Soetikno R, et al. Teleteaching endoscopy: the feasibility of real-time, uncompressed video transmission by using advanced-network technologies. Gastrointest Endosc 2009;70:1013–7.
36. Haycock AV, Youd P, Bassett P, et al. Simulator training improves practical skills in therapeutic GI endoscopy: results from a randomized, blinded, controlled study. Gastrointest Endosc 2009;70:835–45.
37. Koch AD, Buzink SN, Heemskerk J, et al. Expert and construct validity of the Simbionix GI Mentor II endoscopy simulator for colonoscopy. Surg Endosc 2008;22: 158–62.

38. Rex DK. Colonoscopic polypectomy. ASGE Endoscopic Learning Library 2007.
39. Soetikno RM, Barro J, Friedland S, et al. Diagnosis of flat and depressed colorectal neoplasms. ASGE Endoscopic Learning Library 2006.
40. Kudo S. Endoscopic mucosal resection of flat and depressed types of early colorectal cancer. Endoscopy 1993;25:455–61.
41. Kaltenbach T, Friedland S, Maheshwari A, et al. Short- and long-term outcomes of standardized EMR of nonpolypoid (flat and depressed) colorectal lesions > or = 1 cm (with video). Gastrointest Endosc 2007;65:857–65.
42. Monkemuller K, Neumann H, Malfertheiner P, et al. Advanced colon polypectomy. Clin Gastroenterol Hepatol 2009;7:641–52.
43. Hurlstone DP, Karajeh M, Cross SS, et al. The role of high-magnification-chromoscopic colonoscopy in hereditary nonpolyposis colorectal cancer screening: a prospective "back-to-back" endoscopic study. Am J Gastroenterol 2005;100:2167–73.
44. Lynch HT, Smyrk T, Lanspa SJ, et al. Flat adenomas in a colon cancer-prone kindred. J Natl Cancer Inst 1988;80:278–82.

The Importance of the Macroscopic Classification of Colorectal Neoplasms

Yasushi Sano, MD, PhD*, Mineo Iwadate, MD

KEYWORDS

- Colorectal neoplasms • Macroscopic classification
- Non-polypoid colorectal neoplasms • Neoplastic lesions

In Japan, neoplastic lesions of the stomach that have a superficial endoscopic appearance (the lesion appears resectable by endoscopy) are classified as a subtype called "type 0." This term was chosen to distinguish the classification of superficial lesions from Borrmann's classification, proposed in 1926, which described only advanced gastric cancers. This classification method of superficial gastric neoplasia was later applied to the colon and rectum.

The development of the classification of superficial, shallow, depressed-type neoplastic lesions, now classified as 0-IIc, has followed a similar path to that of gastric and early esophageal cancers, but with significant delay. Kariya[1] reported the first 0-IIc lesions in 1977, but until 1993 when Kudo[2] reported the 0-IIc-carcinoma cohort and classification, type 0-IIc carcinomas were thought to be a uniquely Japanese phenomenon. The macroscopic classification of colorectal neoplasms, as defined by the Japanese Society for Cancer of the Colon and Rectum, is shown in **Box 1**. It is essentially identical to that of the gastric superficial neoplasms, with the exception that it does not have type 0-III (the excavated type) because this type does not exist in the colon and rectum.

In 1998, the author's colleagues, Fujii and colleagues,[3] demonstrated the existence and prevalence of 0-IIa and 0-IIc lesions outside Japan in an English population. Saitoh and colleagues[4] and Teixera[5] subsequently reported the incidence of these lesions in a North American and South American population, respectively. By 2003, the importance of the superficial neoplastic lesions in the esophagus, stomach, and colon began to be recognized in Western countries. The development of the Paris classification[6] is important because it provides recognition of the potential importance

Gastrointestinal Center, Sano Hospital, 2-5-1 Shimizugaoka, Tarumi-ku, Kobe, Hyogo, 655-0031, Japan
* Corresponding author.
E-mail address: ys_endoscopy@hotmail.com

Gastrointest Endoscopy Clin N Am 20 (2010) 461–469
doi:10.1016/j.giec.2010.03.014
1052-5157/10/$ – see front matter © 2010 Elsevier Inc. All rights reserved.

> **Box 1**
> **Macroscopic types of primary tumors of the colon and rectum**
>
> Type 0: Superficial tumors
>
>   Type 0-I: Protruded type
>
>   0-Ip: Pedunculated
>
>   0-Isp: Sub-pedunculated
>
>   0-Is: Sessile
>
>   Type 0-II: Superficial type
>
>   0-IIa: Superficial elevated
>
>   0-IIb: Flat type
>
>   0-IIc: Superficial depressed type
>
> Type 1 to 5: Masses with m. propria involvement

of type 0-IIa and 0-IIc and it provides a method for standard classification throughout the world.

The importance and prevalence of the superficial lesions in the colon and rectum caught worldwide public attention in 2008 when Soetikno and colleagues[7] reported the prevalence of non-polypoid (flat and depressed) colorectal neoplasms (NP-CRNs) in asymptomatic and symptomatic adults in North America. The publication put to rest the question of whether or not the flat and depressed colorectal neoplasms exist in Western countries; flat and depressed colorectal neoplasms can be found throughout the world. In this article, the author highlights the importance of the macroscopic classification of the colorectal neoplasm and emphasizes the distinction between so-called flat lesions (IIa and IIb) and superficial depressed (0-IIc) neoplastic colorectal lesions.

BASIC PRINCIPLES
Endoscopic Classification of Superficial Neoplastic Lesions

The Paris endoscopic classification[6] of superficial neoplastic lesions of the digestive tract established a consensus criterion for macroscopic classification of superficial 0-I polypoid and 0-II flat, elevated, and depressed neoplasia. In the colon and rectum, the Paris classification focuses on the degree of protrusion of the lesion, comparing the height of the lesion with that of the closed cups of biopsy forceps (2.5 mm). Lesions protruding above the level of the closed jaws of the biopsy forceps are classified as Is (sessile) lesions; those that are below this level are classified as 0-IIa (elevated); and those at the same level as the forceps (completely flat) are classified as 0-IIb (flat). Regarding depressed lesions, the entire thickness of the neoplasia is located below the level of normal mucosa, resulting in a well-defined, depressed area (0-IIc) (**Figs. 1–3**). A subgroup of superficially elevated lesions (0-IIa) may reach a large lateral diameter (>10 mm) without much increase in height; in the colon, these lesions are called laterally spreading tumors (LST) (**Fig. 4**).[2] In the experiences of the National Cancer Center Hospital, Japan, type 0-IIa comprises nearly half of all type 0 lesions, whereas type 0-IIc, including the combined type, comprises approximately 2%. However, completely flat lesions (0-IIb) are extremely infrequent in contrast with those in the stomach or esophagus (**Fig. 5**).

Using the Paris classification, many small diminutive lesions may be classified as type 0-IIa and one may think that type 0-IIa refers only to the small diminutive lesion.

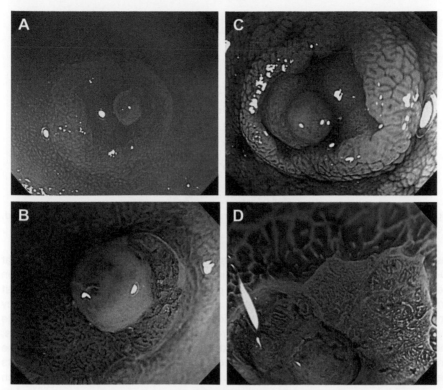

Fig. 1. Various endoscopic imaging of early colon cancer using image enhanced endoscopy. (*A*) Conventional endoscopy. 0-IIc type depressed lesion. (*B*) Optical digital method using narrow band light in image enhanced endoscopy. Capillary pattern type IIIA can be seen on the depressed area. (*C*) Chromoendoscopy contrast method using indigo carmine dye in image enhanced endoscopy. Kudo's type Vi pit pattern can be seen on the depressed area. (*D*) Chromoendoscopy contrast method using crystal violet dye in image enhanced endoscopy. Kudo's type Vi pit pattern can be seen clearly on the depressed area.

In fact, some think that the flat lesion nomenclature describes only these small diminutive lesions. Because diminutive lesions typically do not harbor advanced pathology, the term flat, therefore, may be mistakenly extrapolated as non-important diminutive lesions. The consequence of this assumption is not insignificant. Namely, the studies by Fujii, Teixera, Soetikno, and others showed the existence and important prevalence of the larger type 0-IIa neoplasms, some of these lesions, although large, can be subtle to detect and diagnose, difficult to manage, and have a higher association with advanced pathology compared with polypoid lesions, regardless of size. The large type 0-IIa (LST) includes lesions with a smooth or granular/nodular surface. The smooth surface 0-IIa, which has been described as non-granular, often contains multi-foci of high-grade dysplasia or slightly invasive carcinoma. The granular surface 0-IIa is typically a villous adenoma; if it contains slightly invasive carcinoma, it typically is located in the most protruding granule (ie, the nodule).

The Importance of Distinguishing Between the So-Called Flat Lesion and 0-IIc Type Lesion

Non-protruding or non-polypoid neoplastic lesions are often equated as flat lesions. Note that this is incorrect. Non-protruding or non-polypoid does NOT equate to flat

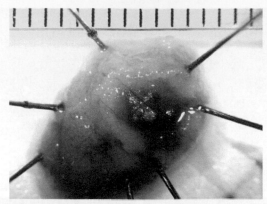

Fig. 2. Resected material under stereomicroscope. En block resection is performed. Depressed lesion, 4 mm in size, can be seen.

lesions alone. Non-polypoid includes the superficial elevated (0-IIa); completely flat (0-IIb); or depressed (0-IIc) lesions. This distinction is important in the classification because in contrast to the high-malignant potential of depressed 0-IIc lesions, most small adenomatous lesions, classified as 0-IIa (**Fig. 6**), do not harbor malignancy and are not clinically significant.[6] In previous reports, the incidence of high-grade dysplasia in so-called flat lesions ranges from 1.78%[9] to 75.0%.[10] In these reports, there was no distinction of the depressed lesions. The significant variation of the finding of high-grade dysplasia or submucosal invasive carcinomas in these reports has perhaps made it difficult for endoscopists to understand what flat lesions mean

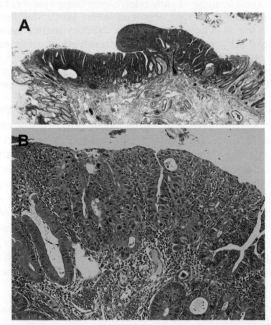

Fig. 3. Histologic findings of resected martial. (*A*) Well-differentiated adenocarcinoma in situ (pM). (*B*) High-power view of the right sided lesion. The glands show structural atypia and their nuclei are hyperchromatic.

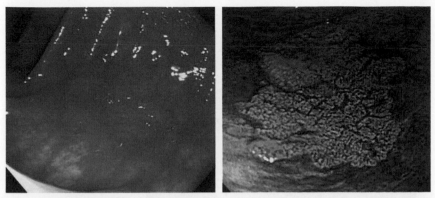

Fig. 4. Laterally spreading tumors. Superficial elevated lesion (0-IIa), so-called laterally spreading tumor (non-granular type) of the transverse colon, 20 mm in diameter. Faint redness in an oval shape with loss of original capillary pattern can be seen (*left*). After spraying dye, a superficial shallow elevated lesion can be clearly identified (*right*). Histologic examination demonstrates well-differentiated adenocarcinoma with submucosal invasion (depth of invasion of the submucosa: sm1, 400 μm).

clinically. Because of the markedly different clinical significance, flat (0-IIa and 0-IIb) and depressed lesions (0-IIc) should be classified and considered separately.[11] Use of umbrella terms, such as non-polypoid or superficial, without understanding the different types of non-polypoid can be misleading and should be used with caution. Thus, the importance of using a standardized classification, such as the Paris standard endoscopic classification[6] of superficial neoplastic lesion, is emphasized.

Distinguishing the Depressed Area of the 0-IIc Neoplastic Lesion

Many small lesions appear to have a slight dimple. Are these lesions classified as IIc (depressed) lesions? As discussed previously, a central depression in the tumor surface is considered to be an important index of the malignant potential of non-polypoid neoplastic lesions. The shape of the edge of the central depression is roughly divided into three types: barnacle type, smooth-edged lake-bed type, and highly

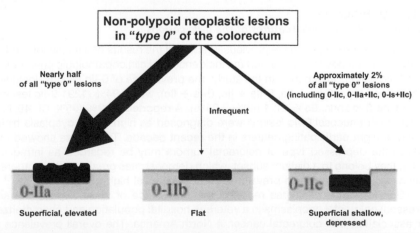

Fig. 5. Endoscopic classification of non-polypoid neoplastic lesions in the colorectum.

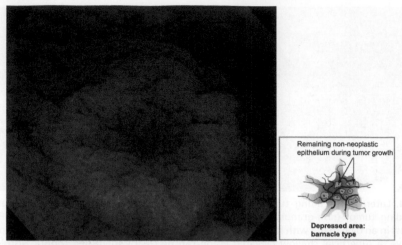

Remaining non-neoplastic
epithelium during tumor growth

Depressed area:
barnacle type

Fig. 6. Small 0-IIa lesion. Small 0-IIa lesion that appears at first glance to have a depression. After dye spraying, some 0-IIa lesions less than 5 mm in diameter show a shallow, ill-defined depression on the surface with groove-like appearance. Sometimes these lesions have a remaining non-neoplastic epithelium on the surface of the lesion.[8] The depression, however, is usually classified as a relatively depressed area, because the depression is still higher than the surface of the adjacent mucosa. Kudo and colleagues used to classify these lesions as 0-IIa with pseudo-depression (IIa + dep), but since Paris, these lesions are classified as 0-IIa because of their lack of malignancy: the incidence of invasive cancer from 0-IIa lesion less than 5 mm is low.

irregular lake-bed type. The barnacle type (see **Fig. 6**) should be distinguished from the latter two types, because it is typically 0-IIa and this lesion type does not correlate with malignancy.[11] However, the latter two types (**Fig. 7**) signify the depressed 0-IIc lesions. These two cases also illustrate the importance of using dye-based image enhancement with diluted indigo carmine solution in the evaluation of the depressed lesions. The irregularity of the boundary of the depression can be clearly visible only after dye spraying and correlates with malignancy.[12]

CLINICAL SIGNIFICANCE
Prevalence and Pathologic Features of the 0-IIc Lesions

The author and colleagues have previously reported the results of a multicenter retrospective cohort study that described the incidence and clinicopathologic characteristics of 0-IIc lesions in Japan.[13] In the study, the prevalence of 0-IIc lesions, including the combined type (0-IIc + IIa, 0-IIa + IIc, 0-Is + IIc), was 1.94% (1291 0-IIc lesions/ 66,670 type 0 lesions, 95% CI: 1.83%–2.04%). A reported 51.2% (95% CI: 49.1%– 54.3%) of intramucosal 0-IIc lesions were diagnosed as high-grade dysplasia histologically at eight participating centers in the recent decade. These data showed that although the depressed type of colorectal tumors may be regarded as infrequent lesions, they belong to a distinct subset, which demonstrates greater biologic aggressiveness according to a high prevalence of intramucosal high-grade dysplasia.[14] In 2008, Soetikno and colleagues reported the prevalence of non-polypoid (flat and depressed) colorectal neoplasms in a veterans hospital population and characterized their association with colorectal cancer in North America. The overall prevalence of NP-CRNs was 9.35%. The overall prevalence of NP-CRNs with in situ or submucosal

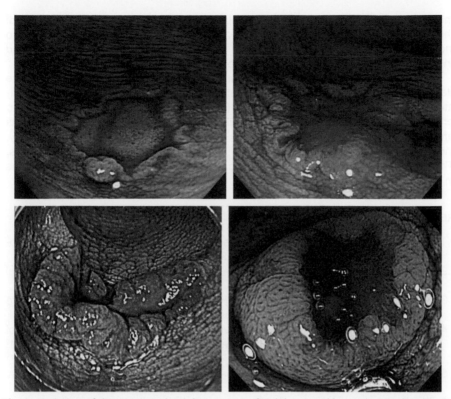

Fig. 7. Variation of the 0-IIc neoplastic lesion. Superficial depressed lesion (0-IIc) of the transverse colon, 8 mm in diameter (*upper left*). After dye spraying, an absolutely depressed area can be clearly identified. Histologic examination demonstrates high-grade dysplasia. Because of the shape of the edge of the central depression, this is classified as a smooth–edged, lake-bed type. Superficial depressed lesion (0-IIc + IIa) (*upper right and lower left*). After dye spraying, an absolutely depressed central area was clearly identified. Histologic examination demonstrates well-differentiated adenocarcinoma with submucosal invasion. Because of the shape of the edge of the central depression, this is classified as a highly irregular lake-bed type. Superficial depressed lesion (0-IIa + IIc) (*lower right*). After dye spraying, an absolutely depressed central area was clearly identified. Histologic examination demonstrates well-differentiated adenocarcinoma with deeper submucosal invasion. Because of the shape of the edge of the central depression, this is classified as a smooth-edged, lake-bed type.

invasive carcinoma was 0.82% (95% CI, 0.46%–1.36%; n = 15). In the screening population the prevalence was 0.32% (95% CI, 0.04%–1.17%; n = 2). Overall, NP-CRNs were more likely to contain carcinoma (odds ratio, 9.78; 95% CI, 3.93–24.4) than polypoid lesions, regardless of the size. The depressed type had the highest risk (33%). NP-CRNs containing carcinomas were smaller in diameter as compared with the polypoid ones (mean [standard deviation] diameter, 15.9 [10.2] mm vs 19.2 [9.6] mm, respectively).[7]

SUMMARY

Without question, the detection, diagnosis, and proper management of IIa, IIb, and IIc lesions in the colon and rectum are important. The classification allows us to stratify the malignant potential of colorectal neoplasms during colonoscopy. Recognition of the existence and importance of NP-CRN is an important first step, but must also incorporate the recognition that NP-CRN includes the superficial elevated/flat and the depressed types, which are distinct from one another.

Further studies are needed to understand the importance and biology of the depressed 0-IIc colorectal tumors. A multicenter randomized controlled trial initiated in 2003, the Japan Polyp Study (JPS), is currently being undertaken to prospectively evaluate follow-up surveillance strategies in Japanese patients after removal of all polyps detected by high-resolution chromoendoscopy, including the removal of non-polypoid (0-IIa, IIb, and IIc) neoplastic lesions. This study may further clarify the significance and natural history of 0-IIc lesions in Japan.[15,16]

REFERENCES

1. Kariya A. A case of early colonic cancer type IIc associated with familial polyposis coli [abstract]. Stomach Intestine 1977;12:1359–64 [in Japanese].
2. Kudo S. Endoscopic mucosal resection of flat depressed type of early colorectal cancer. Endoscopy 1993;25:455–61.
3. Fujii T, Rembacken BJ, Dixon MF, et al. Flat adenomas in the United Kingdom: are treatable cancers being missed? Endoscopy 1998;30:437–43.
4. Saitoh Y, Waxman I, West AB, et al. Prevalence and distinctive biologic features of flat colorectal adenomas in a North American population. Gastroenterology 2001; 120:1657–65.
5. Teixeira CR. Current status of depressed colorectal neoplasia in Latin America. Early Colorectal Cancer 2004;8:57–60.
6. The Paris endoscopic classification of superficial neoplastic lesions: esophagus, stomach, and colon: November 30 to December 1, 2002. Gastrointest Endosc 2003;58:S3–43.
7. Soetikno RM, Kaltenbach T, Rouse RV, et al. Prevalence of nonpolypoid (flat and depressed) colorectal neoplasms in asymptomatic and symptomatic adults. JAMA 2008;299(9):1027–35.
8. Fujimori T, Fujii S, Sano Y, et al. Initial transformed cells of colorectal adenoma: do they occur at the top of the crypt? J Gastroenterol 2002;37:982–4.
9. O'brien MJ, Winawer SJ, Zauber AG, et al. Flat adenomas in the National Polyp Study: is there increased risk for high-grade dysplasia initially or during surveillance? Clin Gastroenterol Hepatol 2004;2(10):905–11.
10. Hart AR, Kudo S, Mackay EH, et al. Flat adenomas exist in asymptomatic people: important implications for colorectal cancer screening programmes. Gut 1998; 43(2):229–31.
11. Kudo S, Kashida H, Tamura T. Early colorectal cancer: flat or depressed type. J Gastroenterol Hepatol 2000;15:S66–70.
12. Terai T, Miwa H, Imai Y, et al. Analysis of the depressed area of small flat depressed-type colorectal tumors as a marker of malignant potential. Gastrointest Endosc 1997;45:412–4.
13. Okuno T, Sano Y, Ohkura Y, et al. Incidence of and clinicopathological characteristics of depressed type lesions: baseline findings of multicenter retrospective cohort study [abstract]. Early Colorectal Cancer 2004;8:21–7 [in Japanese].
14. Sano Y, Tanaka S, Teixeira CR, et al. Endoscopic detection and diagnosis of 0-IIc neoplastic colorectal lesions. Endoscopy 2005;37(3):261–7.

15. Sano Y, Fujii T, Oda Y, et al. A multicenter randomized controlled trial designed to evaluate follow-up surveillance strategies for colorectal cancer: the Japan Polyp Study. Dig Endosc 2004;16:376–8.
16. Matsuda T, Fujii T, Sano Y, et al. Five-year incidence of advanced neoplasia after initial colonoscopy in Japan: a multicenter retrospective cohort study. Jpn J Clin Oncol 2009;39(7):435–42.

Image-Enhanced Endoscopy Is Critical in the Detection, Diagnosis, and Treatment of Non-Polypoid Colorectal Neoplasms

Tonya Kaltenbach, MD*, Roy Soetikno, MD

KEYWORDS

- Colorectal cancer screening • Image-enhanced endoscopy
- Narrow-band imaging • Autofluorescence imaging
- Chromo-endoscopy

Colonoscopy, the most sensitive test used to detect advanced adenoma and cancer, has been shown to prevent colorectal cancer (CRC) when combined with polypectomy.[1] CRC remains the third most commonly diagnosed cancer and the second leading cause of cancer death in men and women in the United States. In 2009, approximately 100,610 colon and 40,870 rectal cancer cases were diagnosed in the United States. In the same year, approximately 49,920 CRC deaths were projected.[2] Regrettably, some newly diagnosed patients with cancer had a clearing colonoscopy before their diagnosis. Rex and colleagues[3] have estimated that approximately 1 in 130 patients who undergo colon cancer screening colonoscopy will develop an interval CRC within 3 years of their clearing colonoscopy, thought mainly to be because of missed or incompletely treated lesions (**Fig. 1**). In the authors' experience, proven fast-growing CRC are thought to be less common (**Fig. 2**).

The knowledge, techniques, and technologies are available today to optimize the colonoscopic detection and diagnosis of pre- or early CRCs, and ultimately, improve advanced CRC prevention. The inconspicuously flat or depressed shape of non-polypoid colorectal neoplasms (NP-CRN), which can cause their detection to

Veterans Affairs Palo Alto Health Care System, 3801 Miranda Avenue, GI-111, Palo Alto, CA 94304, USA
* Corresponding author.
E-mail address: tonya_kolodziejski@yahoo.com

Gastrointest Endoscopy Clin N Am 20 (2010) 471–485
doi:10.1016/j.giec.2010.04.001
1052-5157/10/$ – see front matter. Published by Elsevier Inc.

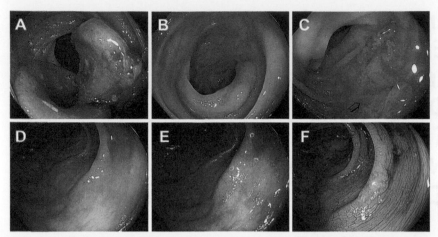

Fig. 1. An interval colon cancer was diagnosed at the hepatic flexure (*A*) during an evaluation for weight loss and iron-deficiency anemia. The patient had a clearing colonoscopy approximately 3 years earlier elsewhere, which was reported to be with good preparation quality. Multiple other, large (*B*) and small (*arrow*) (*C*), superficial elevated (flat) neoplasms were detected. A subtle fourth interval neoplasm—a subcentimeter superficial elevated/flat neoplasm—and its enhanced image using narrow-band imaging and diluted indigo carmine is shown (*D*, *E*, and *F*, respectively).

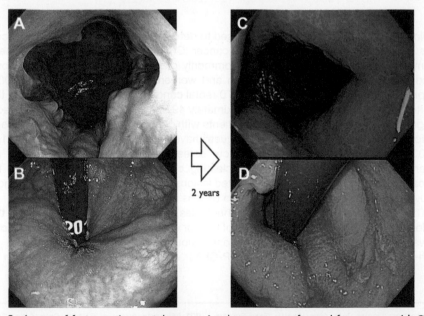

Fig. 2. A case of fast-growing rectal cancer. A colonoscopy performed for average-risk CRC screening 2 years earlier showed the rectum to be normal (*A*, *B*). A subsequent colonoscopy, performed to evaluate symptoms of tenesmus and pain on sitting, showed a large circumferential mass in the distal rectum (*C*, *D*). On endoscopic ultrasound, the lesion was consistent with T3N1. The pathologic condition was signet cell adenocarcinoma. This case also highlights the importance of picture documentation. A picture is worth a thousand words. The lesion was clearly not visible during the examination 2 years previously.

be a challenge, may contribute to interval CRC.[4] Thus, familiarity with subtle mucosal changes in wall contour, color, and vascularity of normal and abnormal mucosa is critical to their successful detection (**Fig. 3**), and a step forward in quality colonoscopy. Image-enhanced endoscopy (IEE) is a useful technique that can be used for detailed inspection and diagnosis of NP-CRN, once an abnormal patch of mucosa has been detected using standard white light colonoscopy.[5] This article reviews the use of IEE in the detection, diagnosis, and treatment of the flat and depressed colorectal neoplasms.

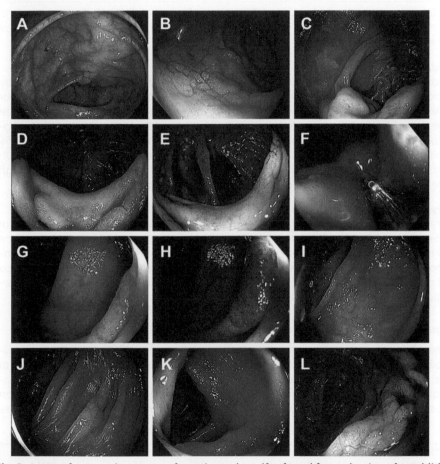

Fig. 3. Images from a colonoscopy of a patient who self-referred for evaluation of a reddish fold (biopsy was adenoma) in the cecum and a large flat adenoma in the transverse colon (*A*). A large flat adenoma in the cecum (*B*) that extended into the ileocecal valve (*C, D*) was diagnosed. The lesion was sprayed with diluted indigo carmine to further delineate its large size, which precluded endoscopic mucosal resection (*E*). Target biopsies were obtained from the area suspected of containing the most advanced pathologic condition (*F*) at the ileocecal valve, and showed adenoma. The patient had multiple other flat adenomas throughout the colon, shown using white light (*G, I, J, K*), NBI (*H*) and indigo carmine (*L*). Note on careful inspection of the still images of these lesions that the lesions seem more reddish compared with the surrounding normal mucosa, have disrupted vascularity, and deformity of the fold contour of the colon wall. Similar to the case shown in **Fig. 1**, these multiple-interval neoplasms suggest that the prior examination was inadequate.

TECHNIQUES OF IMAGE-ENHANCED ENDOSCOPY

IEE can be readily accomplished using dyes or features of the endoscope equipment. In the colon and rectum, dye-based IEE includes the use of indigo carmine and crystal violet, although crystal violet is used primarily in Japan. Endoscope equipment–based IEE is now available through all major gastrointestinal endoscopy manufacturers, with each manufacturer offering a proprietary technique and technology.

Dye-Based IEE Techniques

In the colon and rectum, dye-based IEE includes the use of diluted indigo carmine and crystal violet solutions. These dyes significantly differ in their properties and methods of actions.

Indigo carmine dye

Indigo carmine is a contrast dye, that is, it is not absorbed into the cells. It functions by pooling into the mucosal pits, grooves, erosions, and depressions. Its deep blue color enhances visualization of these structures and allows the endoscopist to characterize the lesions by enabling them to better visualize the border, depth, and surface topography of the lesion. Diluted indigo carmine is usually made by mixing 5 mL of 0.8% solution of indigo carmine (American Reagent Laboratories Inc, Shirley, NY, USA) with 15 mL of water using a 60-mL syringe. The solution is sprayed directly through the accessory channel of the colonoscope (**Table 1**) (**Fig. 4**).

Crystal violet dye

Crystal violet is a vital dye that stains the colonic crypts. It is used by the application of a few drops of 0.1% to 0.5% solution, using a nontraumatic catheter, onto the surface of a lesion to provide a vivid coloration of the pit margins. High-magnification colonoscopy is usually required to best characterize the pit pattern of the lesion. A few drops of crystal violet are used selectively to confirm or to refute the presence of characteristic pit pattern of submucosal invasive carcinoma.

Equipment-Based IEE Techniques

The advent of smaller-sized charge-coupled device cameras (CCDs) permits the availability of high-definition (HD) endoscopy. In turn, HD endoscopy allows visualization of detailed mucosal structures almost to the cellular level. Equipment-based IEE techniques use optical or software technology and are operated by switching a button at the control body of the endoscope. The displayed images are enhanced images

---

Table 1
Preparations of indigo carmine for the detection, diagnosis, and treatment of NP-CRN

1. Solution for image enhancement endoscopy
   4–5 mL of 0.8% indigo carmine mixed with 20 cc water

2. Solution for submucosal injection
   Need: indigo carmine, 19-gauge filter needle, sterile cup (100-mL specimen cup), and 10 mL normal saline flush syringe
   For EMR: Mix 20 drops of indigo carmine using 19-gauge filter needle in 100 mL of sterile normal saline
   For ESD: Mix 1 cc of indigo carmine with 30 cc sterile normal saline
   Mix 1 mL of 1:10,000 Epinephrine in 10 cc of sterile normal saline

Abbreviations: EMR, endoscopic mucosal resection; ESD, endoscopic submucosal dissection.

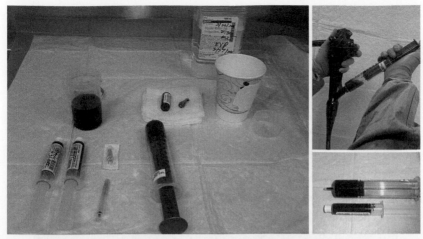

Fig. 4. Use of indigo carmine spray for the detection, diagnosis, and treatment of NP-CRN. One ampoule of 0.8% indigo carmine is used for image enhancement and for submucosal injection (**Table 1**). When a suspicious area that may contain NP-CRN has been identified, or an NP-CRN has been diagnosed, indigo carmine solution made with water for image enhancement is prepared (*left*) using a Luer-lock 60-mL syringe. The solution is sprayed directly through the working channel of the endoscope (*upper right*). In addition, a more diluted solution is made with saline using 10-mL syringes, in preparation for the submucosal injection of the inject-and-cut endoscopic mucosal resection technique. Note the color of the solutions (*lower right*).

obtained through modification of the light source (precapture) or the captured images (postcapture). The general principles of the different technologies are as follows.

Fujinon intelligence color enhancement

Fujinon intelligence color enhancement (FICE), also known as flexible spectral imaging color enhancement, spectral estimation technology, or computed virtual chromoendoscopy, uses a postcapture technology. The reflected light is captured and arithmetically processed into a set of virtual endoscopic images according to a set of narrowed wavelengths, that is, the system computes virtual sets of images that would have been seen had only a narrowed wavelength been used (**Fig. 5**). The system allows the endoscopist to view the enhanced images based on a set of 3 predetermined, empirically chosen, narrowed wavelengths. Up to 10 variable settings are available through settings on the keyboard; the endoscopist selects the setting that best enhances visualization of microvessels, glands, and pits.

Olympus narrow-band imaging

Narrow-band imaging (NBI) uses a precapture equipment-based IEE technology. NBI uses specialized optical filters to modify the white light into narrowed bands of light. Narrowed blue and green lights, with wavelengths centered at 415 and 540 nm, are used, while red light is omitted (**Fig. 6**). The 415 nm wavelength is at the peak light absorption of hemoglobin; thus mucosal microvessels seem dark. In the colon and rectum, microvessels form loops—each loop surrounds an individual gland. Visualization of distorted microvessels enhances the ability to view the distorted neoplastic glands. In addition, the neoplastic process itself induces microvessels to change in configuration, density, and size, thus further allowing the endoscopists to diagnose the condition of the lesion through the endoscope (**Fig. 7**).

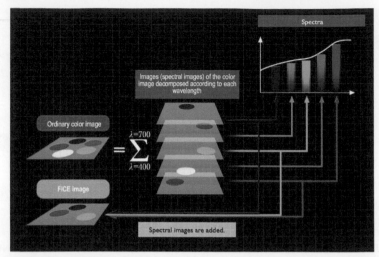

Fig. 5. The principles of FICE.

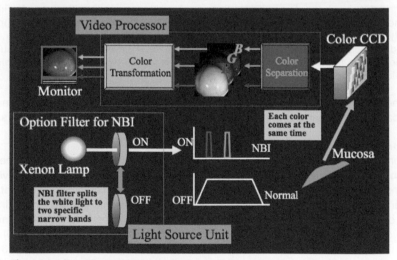

Fig. 6. The principles of narrow-band imaging (NBI) in the color chip system.

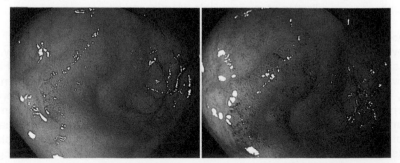

Fig. 7. A superficial elevated (0-IIa) lesion. The mucosal microvessels of the non-polypoid neoplasm seem red in white light (*left*) and dark brown in NBI (*right*).

Olympus autofluorescence imaging

Autofluorescence imaging (AFI) uses a sequential method composed of short wavelengths of blue light (390–470 nm) to excite endogenous fluorophores that then emit green light (540–560 nm). During AFI colonoscopy, nonneoplastic lesions seem green, whereas neoplastic lesions have a longer wavelength emission, appearing magenta (reddish-purple). The AFI colonoscope is equipped with 2 CCDs that can be easily alternated by pushing a button on the scope handle—one standard high-resolution white light and one autofluorescence.

Pentax iScan

The Pentax iScan is a postcapture system that offers 3 types of enhancement: surface enhancement, contrast enhancement, and tone enhancement. The different modalities of iScan enhancement are shown in **Fig. 8**. An additional feature of the iScan includes the twin mode (**Fig. 9**), which provides simultaneous side-by-side viewing of white light and enhanced images.

Principles of Tone Enhancement

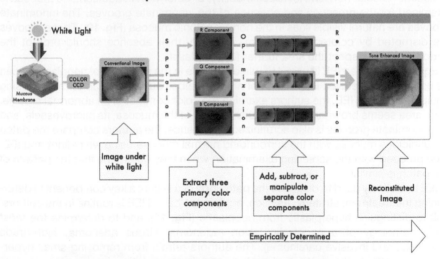

Fig. 8. The principles of the iScan modalities.

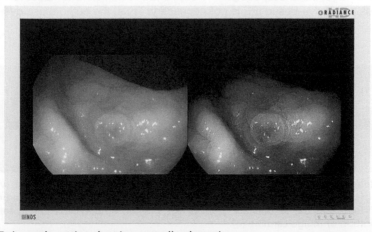

Fig. 9. Twin-mode setting showing a small colon adenoma.

USE OF IEE IN THE COLON AND RECTUM IN THE AUTHORS' PRACTICE

The detection of NP-CRN and the application of IEE require that the mucosa is clean from debris or excess mucus. To detect NP-CRN and to ensure safety of polypectomy, the authors bowel purge using 4 L of polyethylene glycol solution the night before and 1 bottle (296 mL) of magnesium citrate with 1 L of water on the morning of the colonoscopy—in essence creating a split-dose preparation. Patients are allowed to follow a low-residue diet prior to their bowel preparation. In the authors' unit, patients who present with incomplete bowel preparation are prescribed an additional bottle of magnesium citrate and 1 L of water. The authors then perform a same-day colonoscopy, 2 hours following their completion of the solution.

For colorectal neoplasia detection in patients with an average risk for CRC, mucosal examination is initiated using high-resolution or HD white light, and techniques of IEE selectively applied to areas that seem abnormal on white light imaging. The key to the detection of NP-CRN is to search for an abnormal-appearing patch of mucosa, which may contain characteristics of NP-CRN that include a slight red discoloration, altered or absent vascular network, localized friability, or deformity. In addition, the mucosa is examined for the presence and absence of the innominate grooves. The innominate grooves are natural visible lines in the normal colonic mucosa (**Fig. 10**). These grooves are disrupted by colorectal neoplasm. As such, their absence should prompt the endoscopist to inspect the area further for neoplasia.

Equipment-based IEE is useful to rule out or rule in the presence of neoplasm. It can be used to gain detailed information of a subtle, albeit suspicious, abnormality. Using equipment-based IEE, the authors examine the color contrast of an abnormal area (ie, if the area seems browner). The glandular pattern of the mucosa, its microvessels, and the innominate grooves is also scrutinized. In essence, the authors compare the patch of suspicious mucosa with the surrounding normal mucosa using white light and IEE, then proceed with the screening examination when they determine that the pattern of the patch is similar.

IEE is routinely used to diagnose the pathology of a lesion; a key component in determining the treatment strategy. As such, equipment-based IEE is routine in the authors' unit to distinguish hyperplastic from neoplastic (**Fig. 11**), and to determine the most likely pathology of a neoplastic lesion (adenoma, villous adenoma, high-grade dysplasia, and invasive carcinoma). The authors refrain from removing small hyperplastic lesions in the colon and rectum and from resecting invasive carcinomas (**Fig. 12**). In most instances, equipment-based IEE is sufficient for close evaluation of the lesion and dye-based IEE is not necessary. Thus, the authors use dye-based

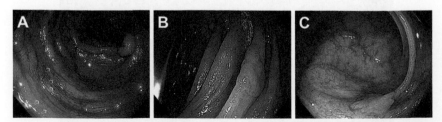

Fig. 10. Innominate grooves. The normal colon-lining appearance is enhanced with the pooling of the indigo carmine dye into the innominate grooves (A). A non-polypoid neoplasm interrupts the innominate grooves (B), and can be best appreciated following the application of indigo carmine (C).

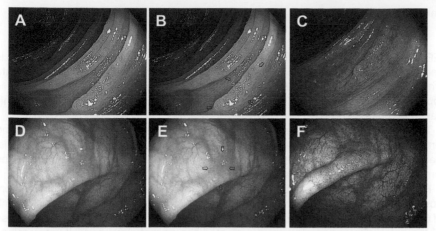

Fig. 11. Diagnostic use equipment-based IEE, to correlate mucosal and microvascular patterns. Closer inspection of a fold irregularity detected on withdrawal using white light (*A, B*) showed a hyperplastic lesion pattern using NBI (*C*); whereas further inspection of a redness patch in white light (*D, E*) revealed an adenomatous microvascular pattern on NBI (*F*).

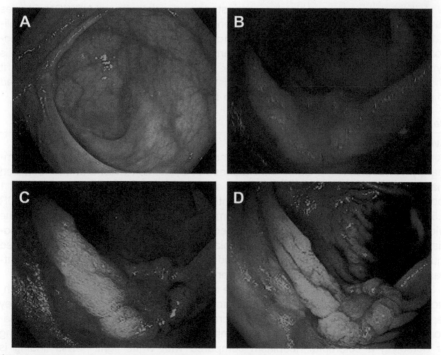

Fig. 12. A 12-mm depressed lesion (IIc) was identified in the cecum near the appendiceal orifice during surveillance colonoscopy (*A*). The patient had a pedunculated villous adenoma with high-grade dysplasia removed from the sigmoid colon 5 years previously. Despite the small size of the lesion, the lesion's features of fold convergence and submucosal fullness on white light were suggestive of massive submucosal invasion (*B*). Inspection with NBI showed a dense irregular microvascular pattern (*C*), and the indigo carmine enhanced the depressed morphology (*D*). In such a case mucosal resection was not attempted, but a targeted biopsy of the depression was obtained that showed adenocarcinoma. The patient had surgery; the study showed submucosal invasive moderately differentiated adenocarcinoma with 1 out of 20 lymph nodes being positive (T1N1).

IEE using indigo carmine solution in cases where further diagnostic information is needed to refine their endoscopic diagnosis. Indigo carmine is also used to evaluate whether an NP-CRN is a depressed lesion by observing the pooling of the dye. This topographic assessment using the dye is often irreplaceable using equipment-based IEE.

The authors do not use methylene blue. Although it also provides a blue coloring similar to indigo carmine, methylene blue is a vital dye and is absorbed into cells. Because of this property methylene blue is not readily washable, and can make the lumen darker and the mucosa seem unpleasantly dirty.

For colorectal neoplasia detection in patients with long-standing inflammatory bowel disease of the colon, the authors use diluted indigo carmine solution (10 mL of 0.4% in 250 mL of water) sprayed using the water jet during the examination phase of the colon. Recent studies have indicated the use of dye-based IEE to replace random biopsy for screening of colorectal neoplasms in patients with chronic ulcerative colitis.

SUPPORTING LITERATURE DATA FOR THE AUTHORS' PRACTICE

White light endoscopy remains the cornerstone to the detection of NP-CRN. Studies have assessed the influence of IEE on adenoma detection. In such studies the application of IEE techniques has been shown to lead to a higher yield in adenoma detection in high-risk groups, including inflammatory bowel disease and polyposis syndrome cohorts, but not in average-risk CRC screening populations. However, it should be noted that no study in the published literature to date has been designed to primarily investigate the effect of IEE on the detection of NP-CRN.

Detection of Colorectal Neoplasia

Average-risk screening

For neoplasia detection in asymptomatic and symptomatic patients, excluding inflammatory bowel disease, a Cochrane Database of Systemic Reviews of 4 randomized trials showed that indigo carmine yielded significantly more patients with at least 1 (odds ratio [OR] 1.61, 95% confidence interval [CI] 1.24–2.09) and 3 or more (OR 2.55, CI 1.49–4.36) neoplastic lesions compared with standard colonoscopy.[6] The widespread clinical application of dye-based IEE to the colon was limited by its association with a high detection rate of hyperplastic lesions and perceptions of obscured mucosal visualization because of the pooled solution.[7–9] The availability of equipment-based IEE was attractive, making a dye spray unnecessary.

Several recent studies have reported the application of equipment-based IEE techniques for adenoma detection. In the authors' NBI tandem colonoscopy study, they reported high adenoma detection rates across screening and nonscreening populations, although they did not find NBI to significantly influence the likelihood of missing or detecting a colorectal neoplasm compared with white light.[10] This finding is complementary to other randomized NBI trials—in the United States by Rex and Helbig,[11] in Japan by Inoue and colleagues,[12] and most recently in Italy by Paggi and colleagues.[13] Pooled results of these trials totaling more than 2000 patients did not show significant differences in adenoma detection between NBI and white light for CRC screening.[14,15] A subgroup analysis, based on lesion morphology, has suggested significantly higher yield of flat adenoma detection with NBI compared with white light examination (OR 2.02, CI 1.51–2.72).[15]

The use of AFI has also been investigated in this setting, albeit on a lesser scale. Using the AFI technology in a modified back-to-back colonoscopy pilot study, a single experienced Japanese endoscopist showed high detection rates of right-sided colonic polyps, especially flat and/or diminutive adenomatous lesions, compared with conventional white light colonoscopy.[16]

The application of the postprocessing technology in the screening colonoscopy population has also recently been investigated. A large, prospective, randomized multitertiary care center trial reported similar adenoma detection properties of FICE compared with conventional colonoscopy with targeted indigo carmine.[17] The use of iScan to improve the detection of NP-CRN has not been reported.

High-risk screening
Ulcerative colitis Most neoplastic and dysplastic lesions in the ulcerative colitis population are non-polypoid,[18] and surveillance colonoscopy with IEE is recommended.[19] Rutter and colleagues[20] showed a higher sensitivity of pancolonic chromoendoscopy with indigo carmine dye spraying for the detection of intraepithelial neoplasias in patients with long-standing ulcerative colitis. During the first conventional examination, visible abnormalities were biopsied, and quadratic nontargeted biopsies were taken every 10 cm. Pancolonic indigo carmine was used during the second colonoscopic examination, and any additional visible abnormalities were biopsied. No dysplasia was detected in 2904 nontargeted biopsies. In comparison, a targeted biopsy protocol with pancolonic chromoendoscopy was more specific—requiring fewer biopsies (n = 157) yet detecting 9 dysplastic lesions. Several other studies have shown similar increases in diagnostic yield of dysplasia using indigo carmine or methylene blue IEE.[21–23]

The use of equipment-based IEE to detect and diagnose neoplasia in ulcerative colitis has recently been reported. One prospective, randomized, crossover study of 42 patients with long-standing ulcerative colitis failed to show superior neoplasia detection rates using NBI compared with conventional colonoscopy.[24] The same research group showed improved detection using targeted biopsy with AFI compared with a lower yield with random biopsies.[25]

Hereditary nonpolyposis colorectal cancer Relative to conventional colonoscopy, the application of IEE significantly improves adenoma detection in patients with hereditary nonpolyposis colorectal cancer (HNPCC) syndrome. Studies showed the efficacy of indigo carmine for improved adenoma detection in the proximal colon in patients with HNPCC, and report significantly higher diagnoses of flat lesions, increasing from 6% before to 24% after chromoendoscopy.[26] East and colleagues[27] examined the adenoma-detection efficacy of NBI in this polyposis surveillance cohort. These investigators performed NBI examination following white light examination on all patients, and concluded that the use of NBI in the proximal colon appeared to improve adenoma detection, especially in non-polypoid lesions. The study design did not incorporate a comparative control (ie, repeat white light examination to assess the NBI effect versus the intrinsic miss rate of colonoscopy). Another back-to-back surveillance colonoscopy study of 109 HNPCC patients reported superiority of indigo carmine (48%; 52/109) in adenoma detection, compared with index white light (15%; 7/47) or NBI (18%; 11/62) colonoscopy—albeit the adenoma detection rates were remarkably low in the white light and NBI examinations.[28]

Diagnosis of Colorectal Lesions

Differentiation of nonneoplastic and neoplastic tissue
Dye-based and equipment-based IEE techniques have been shown to facilitate accurate real-time histopathologic diagnosis of colon lesions. Kudo has been the main

proponent of the use of indigo carmine, coupled with high-magnification colonoscopy, to accurately diagnose colorectal lesions. He described the characteristic pit-pattern morphology of normal, nonneoplastic, and neoplastic colon mucosa in detail.[29] Matsuda and colleagues,[30] using similar equipment and method, have reported the potential of using a less complex classification wherein lesions are classified to distinguish nonneoplasm, mucosal neoplasm, and submucosal invasive neoplasm.

In Western countries, high-magnification colonoscopy with dye-based IEE has not gained popularity and is largely unavailable. As such, efforts have been redirected to the use of HD colonoscopy coupled with equipment-based IEE for real-time endoscopic diagnosis. The early studies of equipment-based IEE have shown high diagnostic accuracy of polyp histology. In a recent comparison of NBI with white light using HD colonoscopes, NBI showed significant superiority for real-time differentiation of nonneoplastic and neoplastic colon polyps.[31] Equipment-based postprocessing IEE is now also under study. A single study in a screening population showed similar diagnostic characteristics of iScan to methylene blue for neoplasia diagnosis in the distal colon.[32]

Real-time differentiation of neoplastic and normal tissue is also an important skill in the endoscopic resection of NP-CRN. IEE with indigo carmine is commonly used in this setting. Immediately following mucosectomy, IEE analysis of the pit and vascular tissue pattern at the resection margins can help identify any residual neoplasia from an incomplete resection. If residual neoplasm is identified, further resection or ablative techniques can be directly applied. Outcomes analysis of endoscopic mucosal resection of flat lesions greater than 2 cm in size showed a reduction of local neoplastic recurrence from 8.7% to 0.5% (P<.01) following the implementation of the routine use of high magnification with IEE in tumor residual assessment.[33] Similarly, IEE is a useful adjuvant technique in surveillance examination to assess the scar site in detail for local recurrence (**Fig. 13**).

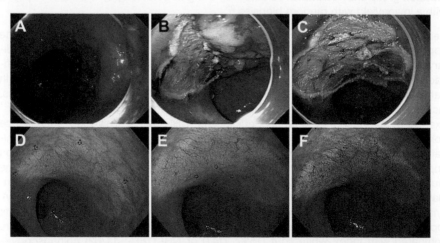

Fig. 13. Close examination of a scar post endoscopic mucosal resection (EMR) showing focal area of local recurrence. The patient had piecemeal EMR using the inject-and-cut technique (*A, B ,C*). Note the use of a slightly tinted saline with indigo carmine to inject the submucosa. Because saline injection into the muscularis propria typically does not stay, the blue tinged tissue is the submucosa. Thus, the resection was in the appropriate layer. Follow-up a few months later (*D*) showed a small area of possible local recurrence (*E, small arrows*). Targeted biopsy of the suspicious area immediately adjacent to the red arrow (*F*) showed adenoma, while the rest of the scar did not show adenoma.

SUMMARY

IEE is an integral part in the detection, diagnosis, and treatment of NP-CRN. Both the dye-based and equipment-based varieties of IEE are readily available for application in today's practice of colonoscopy. Data are available to support its use, although further studies are needed to simplify the classification of colorectal lesions by the different techniques of equipment-based IEE.

REFERENCES

1. Winawer SJ, Zauber AG, Ho MN, et al. Prevention of colorectal cancer by colono-scopic polypectomy. The National Polyp Study Workgroup. N Engl J Med 1993; 329:1977–81.
2. Jemal A, Siegel R, Ward E, et al. Cancer statistics, 2009. CA Cancer J Clin 2009; 59:225–49.
3. Rex DK, Bond JH, Feld AD. Medical-legal risks of incident cancers after clearing colonoscopy. Am J Gastroenterol 2001;96:952–7.
4. Soetikno RM, Kaltenbach T, Rouse RV, et al. Prevalence of nonpolypoid (flat and depressed) colorectal neoplasms in asymptomatic and symptomatic adults. JAMA 2008;299:1027–35.
5. Kaltenbach T, Sano Y, Friedland S, et al. American Gastroenterological Associa-tion (AGA) Institute technology assessment on image-enhanced endoscopy. Gastroenterology 2008;134:327–40.
6. Brown SR, Baraza W, Hurlstone P. Chromoscopy versus conventional endoscopy for the detection of polyps in the colon and rectum. Cochrane Database Syst Rev 2007;4:CD006439.
7. Kiesslich R, von Bergh M, Hahn M, et al. Chromoendoscopy with indigocarmine improves the detection of adenomatous and nonadenomatous lesions in the colon. Endoscopy 2001;33:1001–6.
8. Hurlstone DP, Sanders DS, Cross SS, et al. Colonoscopic resection of lateral spreading tumours: a prospective analysis of endoscopic mucosal resection. Gut 2004;53:1334–9.
9. Brooker JC, Saunders BP, Shah SG, et al. Total colonic dye-spray increases the detection of diminutive adenomas during routine colonoscopy: a randomized controlled trial. Gastrointest Endosc 2002;56:333–8.
10. Kaltenbach T, Friedland S, Soetikno R. A randomised tandem colonoscopy trial of narrow band imaging versus white light examination to compare neoplasia miss rates. Gut 2008;57:1406–12.
11. Rex DK, Helbig CC. High yields of small and flat adenomas with high definition colonoscopes using either white light or narrow band imaging. Gastroenterology 2007;133:42–7.
12. Inoue T, Murano M, Murano N, et al. Comparative study of conventional colono-scopy and pan-colonic narrow-band imaging system in the detection of neoplastic colonic polyps: a randomized, controlled trial. J Gastroenterol 2008;43:45–50.
13. Paggi S, Radaelli F, Amato A, et al. The impact of narrow band imaging in screening colonoscopy: a randomized controlled trial. Clin Gastroenterol Hepatol 2009;7:1049–54.
14. van den Broek FJ, Reitsma JB, Curvers WL, et al. Systematic review of narrow-band imaging for the detection and differentiation of neoplastic and nonneoplas-tic lesions in the colon (with videos). Gastrointest Endosc 2009;69:124–35.
15. Pasha S, Leighton JA, Das A, et al. Narrow Band Imaging (NBI) and White Light Endoscopy (WLE) have a comparable yield for detection of colon polyps in

patients undergoing screening or surveillance colonoscopy: a meta-analysis. Gastrointest Endosc 2009;65:AB363.

16. Matsuda T, Saito Y, Fu KI, et al. Does autofluorescence imaging videoendoscopy system improve the colonoscopic polyp detection rate?—a pilot study. Am J Gastroenterol 2008;103:1926–32.

17. Pohl J, Lotterer E, Balzer C, et al. Computed virtual chromoendoscopy versus standard colonoscopy with targeted indigocarmine chromoscopy: a randomised multicentre trial. Gut 2009;58:73–8.

18. Jaramillo E, Watanabe M, Slezak P, et al. Flat neoplastic lesions of the colon and rectum detected by high-resolution video endoscopy and chromoscopy. Gastrointest Endosc 1995;42:114–22.

19. Farraye FE, Odze RD, Eaden J, et al. AGA technical review on the diagnosis and management of colorectal neoplasia in inflammatory bowel disease. Gastroenterology 2010;138:746–74.

20. Rutter MD, Saunders BP, Schofield G, et al. Pancolonic indigo carmine dye spraying for the detection of dysplasia in ulcerative colitis. Gut 2004;53:256–60.

21. Kiesslich R, Fritsch J, Holtmann M, et al. Methylene blue-aided chromoendoscopy for the detection of intraepithelial neoplasia and colon cancer in ulcerative colitis. Gastroenterology 2003;124:880–8.

22. Hurlstone DP, Sanders DS, Lobo AJ, et al. Indigo carmine-assisted high-magnification chromoscopic colonoscopy for the detection and characterisation of intraepithelial neoplasia in ulcerative colitis: a prospective evaluation. Endoscopy 2005;37:1186–92.

23. Marion JF, Waye JD, Present DH, et al. Chromoendoscopy-targeted biopsies are superior to standard colonoscopic surveillance for detecting dysplasia in inflammatory bowel disease patients: a prospective endoscopic trial. Am J Gastroenterol 2008;103:2342–9.

24. Dekker E, van den Broek FJ, Reitsma JB, et al. Narrow-band imaging compared with conventional colonoscopy for the detection of dysplasia in patients with long-standing ulcerative colitis. Endoscopy 2007;39:216–21.

25. van den Broek FJ, Fockens P, van Eeden S, et al. Endoscopic tri-modal imaging for surveillance in ulcerative colitis: randomised comparison of high-resolution endoscopy and autofluorescence imaging for neoplasia detection; and evaluation of narrow-band imaging for classification of lesions. Gut 2008;57:1083–9.

26. Lecomte T, Cellier C, Meatchi T, et al. Chromoendoscopic colonoscopy for detecting preneoplastic lesions in hereditary nonpolyposis colorectal cancer syndrome. Clin Gastroenterol Hepatol 2005;3:897–902.

27. East JE, Suzuki N, Stavrinidis M, et al. Narrow band imaging for colonoscopic surveillance in hereditary non-polyposis colorectal cancer. Gut 2008;57:65–70.

28. Adler A, Pohl H, Papanikolaou IS, et al. A prospective randomised study on narrow-band imaging versus conventional colonoscopy for adenoma detection: does narrow-band imaging induce a learning effect? Gut 2008;57:59–64.

29. Kudo S. Early colorectal cancer. Tokyo (Japan): Igaku-Shoin; 1996.

30. Matsuda T, Fujii T, Saito Y, et al. Efficacy of the invasive/non-invasive pattern by magnifying chromoendoscopy to estimate the depth of invasion of early colorectal neoplasms. Am J Gastroenterol 2008;103:2700–6.

31. Rex DK. Narrow-band imaging without optical magnification for histologic analysis of colorectal polyps. Gastroenterology 2009;136:1174–81.

32. Hoffman A, Kagel C, Goetz M, et al. Recognition and characterization of small colonic neoplasia with high-definition colonoscopy using i-Scan is as precise as chromoendoscopy. Dig Liver Dis 2010;42:45–50.
33. Tanaka S, Oka S, Chayama K. Endoscopic mucosal resection for superficial early colorectal carcinoma. Indication, choice of method and outcome. Gastroenterol Endosc 2004;46:243–52.

Assessment of Likelihood of Submucosal Invasion in Non-Polypoid Colorectal Neoplasms

Takahisa Matsuda, MD, PhD[a],*,
Adolfo Parra-Blanco, MD, PhD[b], Yutaka Saito, MD, PhD[a],
Taku Sakamoto, MD[a], Takeshi Nakajima, MD, PhD[a]

KEYWORDS

- Non-polypoid colorectal neoplasm • Submucosal cancer
- Lymph node metastasis • Endoscopic diagnosis
- Magnifying chromoendoscopy

Endoscopic mucosal resection (EMR) is indicated to treat intramucosal colorectal carcinoma because the risk of lymph node metastasis is nil.[1,2] Surgery is indicated to treat submucosal invasive cancers (cancer cells invading through the muscularis mucosa into the submucosal layer but not extending into the muscularis propria) because of the 6% to 12% risk of lymph node metastasis.[3–7] However, there is increasing evidence to suggest that lesions with submucosal invasion lower than 1000 μm, without lymphovascular invasion and without poor differentiation, also have a minimal risk of lymph node metastasis[8] and can be cured by EMR alone. It is therefore important to be able to distinguish neoplasms that are candidates for EMR from those that will require surgery, because EMR of lesions containing massive submucosal invasive cancer is associated with the risk of bleeding and perforation and is unlikely to be curative.

Current endoscopes have high-resolution imaging that provides clear, vivid, and detailed features of the detected lesions. When combined with image enhancement, high-magnification endoscopy can provide a detailed analysis of the morphologic architecture of mucosal crypt orifices (ie, pit pattern) in a simple and quick manner.[9,10] As such, magnifying chromoendoscopy has been shown to be effective for the differential

[a] Endoscopy Division, National Cancer Center Hospital, 5-1-1 Tsukiji, Chuo-ku, Tokyo 104-0045, Japan
[b] Department of Gastroenterology, Central University Hospital of Asturias, Celestino Villamil s/n, 33006 Oviedo, Principado de Asturias, Oviedo, Spain
* Corresponding author.
E-mail address: tamatsud@ncc.go.jp

Gastrointest Endoscopy Clin N Am 20 (2010) 487–496
doi:10.1016/j.giec.2010.03.007
1052-5157/10/$ – see front matter © 2010 Elsevier Inc. All rights reserved.

giendo.theclinics.com

diagnosis between colorectal neoplastic and non-neoplastic lesions and determination of the depth invasion of colorectal cancers. The authors highlight methods to assess depth of invasion of non-polypoid colorectal cancers based on a review of the literature and our experience at National Cancer Center Hospital in Japan.

IMPORTANCE OF ESTIMATION OF SUBMUCOSAL INVASION

In Japan, findings of deep submucosal invasion ($\geq$1000 μm), and/or lymphovascular invasion, and/or poorly differentiated adenocarcinoma in the histopathology of an EMR specimen would lead to consideration for surgery. Though lymphovascular invasion and poorly differentiated adenocarcinoma components are impossible to predict before resection, the vertical depth of invasion of submucosal cancers can be estimated based on the morphologic appearance at the time of endoscopy.

However, estimation of submucosal invasion requires more than the measurement of the lesion size. Small colorectal neoplasms are historically believed to have a lower malignancy potential than large ones, and several authors have reported that the malignant potential of early colorectal cancer increases with size.[11–13] Although this observation may be true for adenomatous lesions, the data for submucosally invasive carcinomas are conflicting. In the authors' own large study involving 583 lesions, they found that that small submucosal cancers ($\leq$10 mm, n = 120) had a similarly aggressive behavior and malignant potential as the larger ones (>10mm, n = 463); the risks of lymph node metastasis were similar (small: 11.2%, large: 12.1%, P = .85), lymphovascular invasion (small: 21.7%, large: 27%, P = .23), and poorly differentiated adenocarcinoma components (small: 10%, large: 17.1%, P = .06).[7] They also described that small submucosal cancers were more likely to have non-polypoid growth (NPG) type[14] than the larger lesions (68.3% vs 46.0%, P<.0001). In this retrospective study, the rate of EMR used as an initial treatment was 33.4% (195/583). EMR was more often used to resect the small lesion rather than the large lesion group (51.6% vs 28.7%, P<.0001). However, they were surprised to find that there were no differences in the positive rate of cut margins in both groups (17.7% vs 19.5%, P = .81). This result implies that EMR should not be easily applied to small colorectal lesions when they appear to be submucosally invasive because of its risk of complication and the concept of no-touch isolation.[15]

ESTIMATION OF SUBMUCOSAL INVASION USING BARIUM ENEMA, ENDOSCOPIC ULTRASONOGRAPHY, AND NONLIFTING SIGN
Barium Enema

The superiority of barium enema over colonoscopy is summarized by Tsuji and colleagues[16] as follows: (1) Barium enema is able to describe the shape of the lesion that is difficult for colonoscopy to observe because of its location. (2) In the case of a large lesion in which it is difficult to endoscopically observe the whole lesion, barium enema can describe the entire shape of the lesion and obtain information on the oral side more easily. (3) The size and location of lesions can be assessed more objectively. (4) The degree of deformity of the lateral view enables the clinician to diagnose the depth of invasion more easily.

The authors retrospectively compared the diagnostic accuracy of colonoscopy and barium enema for submucosal colorectal cancers at 2 National Cancer Centers (Tokyo, Kashiwa) in 2001.[17] One hundred eighty-six (polypoid [Ip, Is]: 117, non-polypoid [IIa, IIa+IIc, IIc, laterally spreading tumor (LST)]: 69) lesions were examined in this study, and the authors investigated the accuracy rate of the lesion's depth by 2 modalities (**Fig. 1**). The colonoscopic accuracy rate was superior to that of the barium enema study

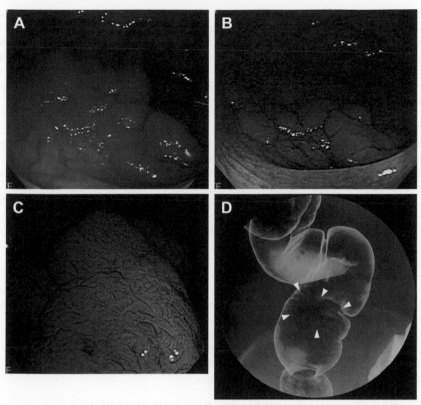

Fig. 1. (*A*) Conventional view, (*B*) Conventional view with indigo carmine dye, (*C*) Magnifying view with crystal violet staining, (*D*) Barium enema image.

(80.1% vs 69.7%, $P = .04$). This result is obtained not only in polypoid lesions (71.8% vs 60.3%, $P = .09$) but also in non-polypoid colorectal lesions (94.2% vs 83.7%, $P = .07$). As a result, the authors concluded that it is sufficient to diagnose the depth of endoscopic resectable early colorectal cancer by colonoscopy alone. However, when selecting surgical management, barium enema or computed tomographic colonography should also be performed to precisely delineate the location of the lesion.

Endoscopic Ultrasonography

Data on the utility of high-frequency endoscopic ultrasonography (EUS) in the management of the malignant colorectal polyp are conflicting. Some authors have reported the usefulness of EUS, particularly the advantages of high-frequency ultrasound (HFUS) to diagnose the invasion depth of early colorectal cancer.[18–21] Hurlstone and colleagues[20] conducted a prospective study to compare the 2 modalities (HFUS vs magnifying chromoendoscopy). They found that HFUS was superior to magnifying chromoendoscopy for determination of depth invasion (93% vs 59% accuracy, respectively [$P<.0001$]). Matsumoto and colleagues[21] also concluded that the negative predictive value of probe-EUS for deep invasion was higher than that of magnifying chromoendoscopy (90.9% vs 54.1%, respectively [$P<.01$]) in the population studied (prevalence deep submucosal invasion 56%).

In contrast, Fu and colleagues[22] have recently reported that magnifying chromoendoscopy is as accurate as EUS for preoperative staging of early colorectal cancer (87% vs 75%, P = .0985). Subgroup analysis was also done for polypoid and nonpolypoid lesions. For polypoid lesions, the respective overall diagnostic accuracies of magnifying colonoscopy and EUS were 88% and 72% (P = .0785), and for nonpolypoid lesions, 85% and 79% (P = .7169). HFUS requires additional training and equipment and can be time-consuming to use.

Nonlifting Sign

Observation of the lesion during and after submucosal saline injection is a simple but important method to assess the potential for deeply invasive cancer. Lesions may not lift because of desmoplastic reaction, invasion from the lesion itself, or submucosal fibrosis from prior biopsy, cautery, ink injection for marking, or ulceration.

Several studies have reported the diagnostic operating characteristics of the nonlifting sign: the positive predictive value of the nonlifting sign is approximately 80%. Originally, Uno and colleagues[23] described this terminology in 1994. Kobayashi and colleagues[24] also reported the verification of the nonlifting sign as one modality of depth diagnosis for colorectal cancers. The nonlifting sign had a sensitivity of 61.5%, a specificity of 98.4%, a positive predictive value of 80%, a negative predictive value of 96%, and an accuracy of 94.8%. In contrast, endoscopic diagnosis using magnifying chromoendoscopy of deeper infiltration had a sensitivity of 84.6%, a specificity of 98.8%, a positive predictive value of 88%, a negative predictive value of 98.4%, and an accuracy of 97.4%. Statistically significant differences were found in terms of sensitivity (P = .031) and accuracy (P = .039). In spite of the simplicity of such a technique, nonlifting sign could not reliably predict deeper cancerous invasion when compared with endoscopic diagnosis.

ESTIMATION OF SUBMUCOSAL INVASION USING CONVENTIONAL AND MAGNIFYING CHROMOENDOSCOPY
Conventional Colonoscopy

New diagnostic modalities such as endoscopic ultrasonography using miniprobe and magnifying chromoendoscopy are reported to be useful for the depth diagnosis of early colorectal cancers. However, these modalities are relatively expensive and time-consuming. Therefore, if invasion depth could be diagnosed with only conventional colonoscopy, it would be more cost-effective and convenient.

Saitoh and colleagues[25] reported that characteristic colonoscopic findings obtained by a combination of videocolonoscopy and chromoendoscopy are clinically useful for determination of the invasion depth of depressed-type colorectal cancers. In this report, characteristic colonoscopic findings, (ie, [1] expansion appearance, [2] deep depression surface, [3] irregular bottom of depression surface, and [4] folds converging toward the tumor) are needed for surgical operation. According to their results, the invasion depth of depressed-type early colorectal cancers could be correctly determined in 58 of 64 lesions (91%) by using these findings.

Data from National Cancer Center Hospital, Tokyo

To clarify the clinically important characteristic colonoscopic findings, the authors reviewed all conventional colonoscopic images of non-polypoid submucosal colorectal cancers treated endoscopically or surgically between 1999 and 2003. There were 123 non-polypoid submucosal colorectal cancers (IIa, LST: 34; IIc, IIa+IIc, Is+IIc [NPG type]: 89) as shown in **Table 1**. In this retrospective review, 7 characteristic colonoscopic findings, (1) tumor size, (2) white spots (chicken-skin appearance), (3)

Table 1
Clinicopathologic characteristics of non-polypoid submucosal cancers

	IIa, LST	IIc, IIa+IIc, Is+IIc
Number of lesions	34	89
Tumor size (mean±SD, mm)	25.4±18.2	15.3±6.8
Histopathologic diagnosis		
SM-superficial (<1000 µm)	19 (56%)	16 (18%)
SM-deep (≥1000 µm)	15 (44%)	73 (82%)
Location		
Right colon	14 (41%)	31 (35%)
Left colon	9 (27%)	23 (26%)
Rectum	11 (32%)	35 (39%)

Abbreviation: SM, submucosal.

redness, (4) firm consistency, (5) expansion, (6) fold convergence, and (7) deep depressed area (**Fig. 2**), were evaluated for association with submucosal deep invasion and then compared with histopathologic results.

Among all the non-polypoid submucosal colorectal cancers, white spots (chicken-skin appearance), redness, firm consistency, and deep depressed area were significantly associated with an increased risk of submucosal deep invasion according to univariate analysis (**Table 2**).

Magnifying Chromoendoscopy

Magnifying chromoendoscopy is a standardized validated method that facilitates detailed analysis of the morphologic architecture of colonic mucosal crypt orifices (pit pattern) in a simple and efficient manner. However, magnifying colonoscopes are still rarely used in endoscopy units. Unrecognized necessity and lack of

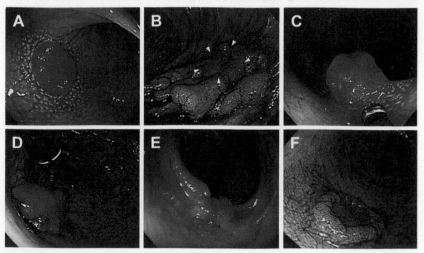

Fig. 2. Six characteristic colonoscopic findings: (*A*) white spots (chicken-skin appearance), (*B*) redness, (*C*) firm consistency, (*D*) expansion, (*E*) fold convergence, and (*F*) deep depressed area.

Table 2
Relationship between endoscopic findings and submucosal deep invasion

	SM-Superficial (n = 35)	SM-Deep (n = 88)	Univariate Analysis (P value)	Diagnostic Sensitivity and Specificity
Size (≥ 20 mm)	16/35 (45.7%)	30/88 (34.1%)	0.23	Sens. 34.1% Spec. 54.3%
White spots (chicken skin) (+)	2/35 (5.7%)	29/88 (32.9%)	0.002	Sens. 32.9% Spec. 94.3%
Redness (+)	14/35 (40.0%)	62/88 (70.4%)	0.002	Sens. 70.4% Spec. 60.0%
Firm consistency (+)	11/35 (31.4%)	69/88 (78.4%)	<0.0001	Sens. 78.4% Spec. 68.6%
Expansion (+)	2/35 (5.7%)	18/88 (20.4%)	0.07	Sens. 20.4% Spec. 94.3%
Fold convergence (+)	4/35 (11.4%)	20/88 (22.7%)	0.24	Sens. 22.7% Spec. 88.6%
Deep depression (+)	15/35 (42.9%)	70/88 (79.5%)	<0.0001	Sens. 79.5% Spec. 57.1%

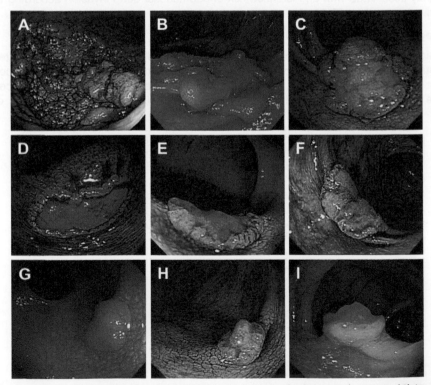

Fig. 3. Representative conventional colonoscopic images of submucosal cancers. (*A*) Is+IIa (LST-granular), (*B*) IIa (LST-nongranular [NG]), (*C*) IIa+IIc (LST-NG), (*D*) IIc, (*E-G*) IIa+IIc, (*H*, *I*) Is+IIc.

randomized studies validating the effectiveness of magnifying chromoendoscopy are possible reasons for this. The authors believe that magnifying chromoendoscopy is essential armamentarium in gastrointestinal endoscopy units and that its main clinical significance is the in vivo diagnosis of the nature of colorectal lesions to determine the appropriate treatment modality.

The clinical classification of the colonic pit pattern (invasive and noninvasive) using magnifying chromoendoscopy was originally described by Fujii in 1998 with the aim to discriminate between intramucosal-submucosal superficial invasion and submucosal deep invasion.[26] Contrary to the anatomic classification by Kudo and colleagues, the rationale for the clinical classification is based on the identification of irregular or distorted crypts in a demarcated area (**Fig. 3**), which strongly suggests that the cancerous lesion is already invading deeply into the submucosal layer.

Some studies have already reported the clinical usefulness of detailed determination of the V pit pattern using magnifying chromoendoscopy for predicting the depth of invasion of submucosal cancers. Kudo and colleagues[10] reported that 11 of 22 (50%) lesions having a type V pit pattern with a bounded surface were found to be invasive cancers with involvement of the submucosal layer. Other studies have reported a diagnostic accuracy of type V pit for the diagnosis of submucosally invasive cancer of 85% (81/95) and 79% (11/14), respectively.[27,28] The authors recently performed a large prospective study of 4215 lesions in 3029 consecutive patients between 1998 and 2005. All lesions were detected by conventional endoscopic view and assessed using magnifying chromoendoscopy for evidence of invasive

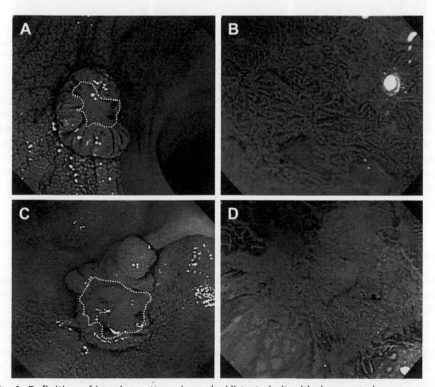

Fig. 4. Definition of invasive pattern: irregular/distorted pit with demarcated area.

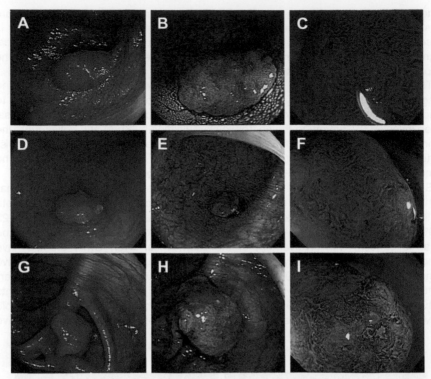

Fig. 5. Submucosal deep cancers. (*A-B*) Is-type submucosal cancer, conventional view. (*C*) Magnifying view (invasive pattern). (*D, E*) IIa+IIc-type submucosal cancer, conventional view. (*F*) Magnifying view (invasive pattern). (*G, H*) Is+IIc-type submucosal cancer, conventional view. (*I*) Magnifying view (invasive pattern).

features according to pit-pattern evaluation. Their data showed that 99.4% of lesions diagnosed as noninvasive pattern were adenoma, intramucosal cancer, or submucosal invasion less than 1000 μm. Among lesions diagnosed with invasive pattern, 87% were cancers with submucosal deep invasion (**Figs. 4** and **5**). Based on the macroscopic appearance, the diagnostic sensitivity of the clinical pit pattern to determine the depth of invasion of polypoid, flat, and depressed lesions was 75.8%, 85.7%, and 98.6%, respectively. This is the first large-scale prospective study to validate the use of magnifying chromoendoscopy as a highly effective method in the prediction of invasion depth of colorectal neoplasms.[29]

SUMMARY

Although of lower prevalence compared with polypoid neoplasms, the non-polypoid neoplasms, especially the depressed type, are important to diagnose because they belong to a distinct biologically aggressive subset, given the high rate of intramucosal or submucosal cancers. The detection and diagnosis of the non-polypoid colorectal neoplasm presents a challenge and an opportunity. Above all, characteristic colonoscopic findings obtained by a combination of conventional colonoscopy and magnifying chromoendoscopy are useful for determination of the invasion depth of non-polypoid colorectal cancers, an essential factor in selecting a treatment modality.

REFERENCES

1. Morson BC, Whiteway JE, Jones EA, et al. Histopathology and prognosis of malignant colorectal polyps treated by endoscopic polypectomy. Gut 1984;25: 437–44.
2. Fujimori T, Kawamata H, Kashida H. Precancerous lesion of the colorectum. J Gastroenterol 2001;36:587–94.
3. Kyzer S, Begin LR, Gordon PH, et al. The care of patients with colorectal polyps that contain invasive adenocarcinoma. Cancer 1992;70:2044–50.
4. Minamoto T, Mai M, Ogino T, et al. Early invasive colorectal carcinomas metastatic to the lymph node with attention to their nonpolypoid development. Am J Gastroenterol 1993;88:1035–9.
5. Cooper HS. Surgical pathology of endoscopically removed malignant polyps of the colon and rectum. Am J Surg Pathol 1983;7:613–23.
6. Nusko G, Mansmann U, Partzsch U, et al. Invasive carcinoma in colorectal adenomas: multivariate analysis of patient and adenoma characteristics. Endoscopy 1997;29:626–31.
7. Matsuda T, Saito Y, Fujii T, et al. Size does not determine the grade of malignancy of early invasive colorectal cancer. World J Gastroenterol 2009;15:2708–13.
8. Participants in the Paris Workshop The Paris endoscopic classification of superficial neoplastic lesions: esophagus, stomach, and colon. November 30 to December 1, 2002. Gastrointest Endosc 2003;58:S3–43.
9. Kudo S, Hirota S, Nakajima T, et al. Colorectal tumours and pit pattern. J Clin Pathol 1994;47:880–5.
10. Kudo S, Tamura S, Nakajima T, et al. Diagnosis of colorectal tumorous lesions by magnifying endoscopy. Gastrointest Endosc 1996;44:8–14.
11. Tanaka S, Yokota T, Saito D, et al. Clinicopathologic features of early rectal carcinoma and indications for endoscopic treatment. Dis Colon Rectum 1995;38:959–63.
12. Saito Y, Fujii T, Kondo H, et al. Endoscopic treatment for laterally spreading tumors in the colon. Endoscopy 2001;33:682–6.
13. Uraoka T, Saito Y, Matsuda T, et al. Endoscopic indications for endoscopic mucosal resection of laterally spreading tumours in the colorectum. Gut 2006; 55:1592–7.
14. Shimoda T, Ikegami M, Fujisaki J, et al. Early colorectal carcinoma with special reference to its development de novo. Cancer 1989;64:1138–46.
15. Wiggers T, Jeekel J, Arends JW, et al. No-touch isolation technique in colon cancer: a controlled prospective trial. Br J Surg 1988;75:409–15.
16. Tsuji Y, Tsuruta O, Miyazaki S, et al. Is it possible to omit barium enema in the diagnosis of advanced colorectal cancer? [abstract]. Endoscopia Digestiva 2001;13: 89–95 [in Japanese].
17. Matsuda T, Fujii T, Saito Y, et al. A comparison of colonoscopy and barium enema for the diagnosis of colorectal cancer with submucosal invasion [abstract]. Endoscopia Digestiva 2001;13:81–7 [in Japanese].
18. Saitoh Y, Obara T, Einami K, et al. Efficacy of high-frequency ultrasound probes for the preoperative staging of invasion depth in flat and depressed colorectal tumors. Gastrointest Endosc 1996;44:34–9.
19. Tsuruta O, Kawano H, Fujita M, et al. Usefulness of the high-frequency ultrasound probe in pretherapeutic staging of superficial-type colorectal tumours. Int J Oncol 1998;13:677–84.
20. Hurlstone DP, Brown S, Cross SS, et al. High magnification chromoscopic colonoscopy or high frequency 20 MHz mini probe endoscopic ultrasound staging for

early colorectal neoplasia: a comparative prospective analysis. Gut 2005;54: 1585–9.

21. Matsumoto T, Hizawa K, Esaki M, et al. Comparison of EUS and magnifying colonoscope for assessment of small colorectal cancers. Gastrointest Endosc 2002;56:354–60.

22. Fu KI, Kato S, Sano Y, et al. Staging of early colorectal cancers: magnifying colonoscopy versus endoscopic ultrasonography for estimation of depth of invasion. Dig Dis Sci. 2007;53:1886–92.

23. Uno Y, Munakata A. The non-lifting sign of invasive colon cancer. Gastrointest Endosc 1994;40:485–9.

24. Kobayashi N, Saito Y, Sano Y, et al. Determining the treatment strategy for colorectal neoplastic lesions: endoscopic assessment or the non-lifting sign for diagnosing invasion depth? Endoscopy 2007;39:701–5.

25. Saitoh Y, Obara T, Watari J, et al. Invasion depth diagnosis of depressed type early colorectal cancers by combined use of videoendoscopy and chromoendoscopy. Gastrointest Endosc 1998;48:362–70.

26. Fujii T, Hasegawa RT, Saitoh Y, et al. Chromoscopy during colonoscopy. Endoscopy 2001;33:1036–41.

27. Kato S, Fujii T, Koba I, et al. Assessment of colorectal lesions using magnifying colonoscopy and mucosal dye-spraying: Can significant lesions be distinguished? Endoscopy 2001;33:306–10.

28. Bianco MA, Rotondano G, Marmo R, et al. Predictive value of magnification chromoendoscopy for diagnosing invasive neoplasia in nonpolypoid colorectal lesions and stratifying patients for endoscopic resection or surgery. Endoscopy 2006;38:470–6.

29. Matsuda T, Fujii T, Saito Y, et al. Efficacy of the invasive/non-invasive pattern by magnifying chromoendoscopy to estimate the depth of invasion of early colorectal neoplasms. Am J Gastroenterol 2008;103:2700–6.

Dynamic Submucosal Injection Technique

Roy Soetikno, MD*, Tonya Kaltenbach, MD

KEYWORDS

• Static submucosal injection • Dynamic submucosal injection
• Endoscopic mucosal resection • Submucosal bleb

Submucosal injection is an integral part of most endoscopic mucosal resection (EMR) techniques. Rosenberg[1] in the United States first described the use of submucosal injection in 1955, using a rigid needle passed through a rigid sigmoidoscope for the purpose of decreasing through and through coagulation of the colonic wall. He was concerned that through-and-through coagulation might lead to injury of the surrounding organ, delayed bleeding, "when separation of too deep a slough uncovers a blood vessel of large size"; intestinal obstruction due to adhesion that formed over a coagulated area; and peritonitis, when the necrotic area is adjacent to the peritoneum.

Deyhle and colleagues[2] in Germany applied the described principles of submucosal injection as a method for flexible endoscopic electroresection of sessile colonic polyp in 1973. After testing the concept in a canine model, they were the first to describe the safety of injecting saline through a flexible injection needle before endoscopic resection of 7 sessile colonic polyps. The submucosal injection technique has since become an integral part of endoscopic mucosal resection[3] and submucosal dissection techniques.[4] In addition, the submucosal injection technique has been applied in the treatment of gastrointestinal bleeding to inject sclerosant or diluted epinephrine to treat variceal[5] and nonvariceal bleeding, respectively, and in marking using India ink or carbon particles.

This article describes the submucosal injection technique applied in the endoscopic resection of non-polypoid colorectal neoplasms, with an emphasis on a particular technique that the authors routinely use in their practice-the dynamic submucosal injection technique.

THE STATIC SUBMUCOSAL INJECTION TECHNIQUE

The technique used to inject the submucosa for endoscopic resection has changed little since the early descriptions. During standard submucosal injection (in this article, the authors propose the term *static submucosal injection technique*), the needle, after being pushed into the submucosa, is kept stationary until an adequate volume of injection has been slowly infused. The lumen is kept fully insufflated to visualize the position

Veterans Affairs Palo Alto Health Care System, 3801 Miranda Avenue, GI-111, Palo Alto, CA 94304, USA
* Corresponding author.
E-mail address: soetikno@earthlink.net

Gastrointest Endoscopy Clin N Am 20 (2010) 497–502
doi:10.1016/j.giec.2010.03.008
1052-5157/10/$ – see front matter. Published by Elsevier Inc.

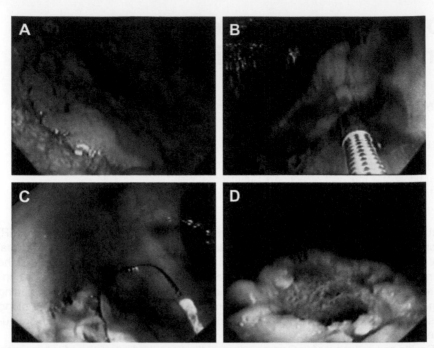

Fig. 1. Static or stationary submucosal injection technique. A 14-mm flat adenoma in the rectum that was resected in the authors' unit in 2000. (*A*) The injection was performed with the needle kept stationary. (*B*) The lesion lifted slightly and a specialized barbed snare was used to capture the lesion. (*C*) The site of resection showed a deep cut. (*D*) The patient had delayed bleeding a few days later.

of the needle. During resection of a large lesion, injection is recommended to begin at the site away from the endoscope. A common disappointment in performing the static submucosal injection technique is that the bulge is insufficient for capturing the lesion by the snare. In these cases, many endoscopists report that the injectant dissipates too fast (**Fig. 1**) and then the snare cannot effectively capture the targeted lesion. Of the several different solutions that have been described to create a larger bulge, only Glyceol (a hypertonic solution consisting of 10% glycerol and 5% fructose in normal saline solution) and hyaluronate are commonly used in Japan.

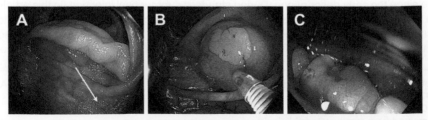

Fig. 2. A simple dynamic submucosal injection. The lesion was partially hidden under a fold. (*A*) The injection was begun with the needle pulled into the endoscope while the tip of the endoscope was pushed slightly downward. (*B*) The path of the needle is shown by the arrow in (*A*). A generous submucosal bleb was formed (*C*).

THE DYNAMIC SUBMUCOSAL INJECTION TECHNIQUE

The authors developed the dynamic submucosal injection technique to facilitate the formation of a massive bulge under the lesion using saline solution and a standard sclerotherapy needle to perform a safe and effective endoscopic mucosal resection and submucosal dissection. To begin, the catheter is engaged at the targeted site of injection, the needle is then exposed into the submucosal, and a small amount (0.5 to 1 mL) of saline is injected to confirm that the tip of the needle is in the submucosa. Subsequent injection is performed through the 25-gauge needle rapidly, but rather than being static, the needle is moved within the injection site by pulling the catheter back slowly or by slightly deflecting the tip of the endoscope. The lumen is suctioned—occasionally to the point of collapse—to increase the size of the bulge. The shape of the submucosal accumulation of the saline is, therefore, molded so that the submucosal bleb raises the flat lesion and then can be easily resected. In EMR cases, the lesion is then resected en-bloc or piecemeal using a commercially available stiff snare. The authors use the technique routinely in practice (representative images are shown in **Figs. 2–6**).

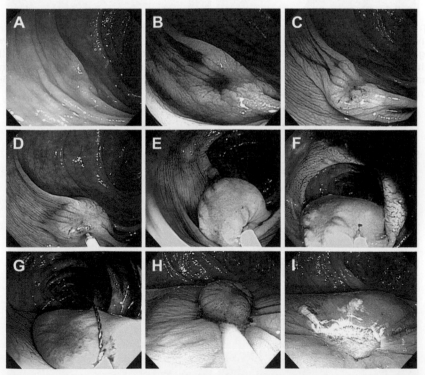

Fig. 3. A 12-mm superficial depressed lesion under white light (*A*) with diluted indigo carmine solution (*B*) and with the lumen slightly deflated (*C*). Dynamic submucosal injection with saline solution was begun (*D*). The lesion began to lift with a rapid injection (*E*), and the needle was raised up and pulled slightly toward the colonoscope while the injection was continued (*F*). There was a localized large bleb under the lesion. The snare was positioned to capture the lesion en-bloc (*G*). The snare was pushed downward (*H*) while the lumen was slightly deflated. The lesion was captured and the resection site showed a complete 1-piece resection (*I*).

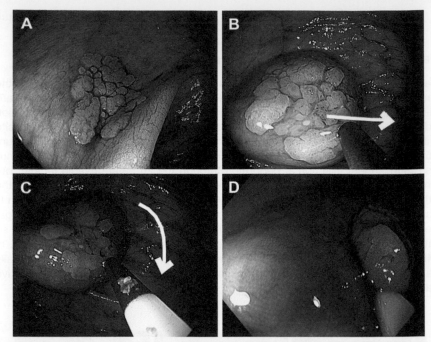

Fig. 4. A 14-mm superficial elevated (flat) lesion after diluted indigo carmine solution (*A*). Dynamic submucosal injection using saline was performed before EMR. The injection was begun at the periphery of the lesion; the tip of the endoscope was moved slightly to the right (*B*) and then downward (*C*), with the lumen was slightly deflated. A generous submucosal bleb was present under the lesion for safe and effective en-bloc mucosal resection using a 10-mm braided snare (*D*).

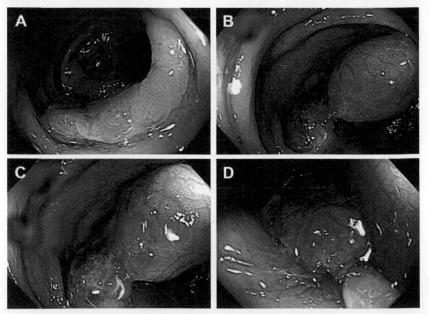

Fig. 5. EMR of a previously attempted polypectomy of a flat lesion (*A*) is difficult because of underlying scar. The appearance of the lesion during dynamic submucosal injection (*B*) using saline. While the lumen was slightly deflated, the needle was lifted toward the opposite wall (*C*). Injection was performed rapidly and the bleb was formed in such a way that the lesion became slightly tilted toward the endoscope. After a thick submucosal cushion had been formed under lesion, the lesion was captured using a stiff braided snare (*D*).

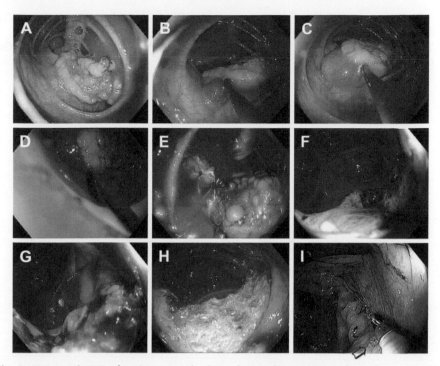

Fig. 6. Piecemeal EMR of a giant granular lateral spreading tumor at the cecum/ascending colon junction (*A*). The case provides an example that manipulation of the needle during the first injection caused the injectant to accumulate in the part of the lesion further away from endoscope, which in turn led the lesion to become tilted toward the endoscope. In this case, while the injection using saline was rapidly performed, the needle was raised up (*B*), the needle was then pulled slightly, and the tip was moved downward (*C, D*). The needle was then kept pushed down while the submucosa was injected. Further injections were then performed surrounding the lesion. Resection was then begun at the periphery (*E*). Inspection of the resection site following the piecemeal snaring showed a small amount of residual tumor. We resect (as opposed to ablate) all visible neoplasia at the time of resection. Thus, we repeated injection using the same dynamic technique – in this case, while lifting the needle upward (*F*). The residue was completely snared (*G*), and then argon plasma coagulation was appiled to the resection margins and exposed superficial vessels (*H*). During the one-year follow-up, there was diminutive (2 mm) adenoma that we removed (*I*) (*thick arrow*).

In conclusion, the dynamic submucosal injection technique is useful to mold an ample submucosal bleb. The bleb, in turn, permits endoscopic resection to be performed safely and efficaciously.

REFERENCES

1. Rosenberg N. Submucosal saline wheal as safety factor in fulguration or rectal and sigmoidal polypi. AMA Arch Surg 1955;70(1):120–2.
2. Deyhle P, Largiader F, Jenny S, et al. A method for endoscopic electroresection of sessile colonic polyps. Endoscopy 1973;5:38–40.
3. Soetikno R, Gotoda T, Nakanishi Y, et al. Endoscopic mucosal resection. Gastrointest Endosc 2003;37:128–32.

4. Saito Y, Sakamoto T, Fukunaga S, et al. Endoscopic submucosal dissection (ESD) for colorectal tumors. Dig Endosc 2009;21(Suppl 1):S7–12.
5. Yeh RW, Triadafilopoulos G. Injection therapies for nonbleeding disorders of the GI tract. Gastrointest Endosc 2006;64(3):399–411.

Endoscopic Mucosal Resection of Non-Polypoid Colorectal Neoplasm

Tonya Kaltenbach, MD*, Roy Soetikno, MD

KEYWORDS

- Non-polypoid colorectal neoplasm
- Endoscopic mucosal resection
- Surveillance colonoscopy • Inject-and-cut technique

Endoscopic mucosal resection (EMR), rather than standard polypectomy, is the preferred resection method of non-polypoid lesions because these lesions can be technically difficult to capture with a snare; furthermore, without submucosal injection the underlying muscularis propria may be excessively coagulated or even inadvertently resected.[1] In addition, because the resection plane of EMR is in the middle or deeper part of the submucosa, EMR allows the precise depth of the lesion to be evaluated. Although the majority of non-polypoid lesions are adenomatous, non-polypoid colorectal neoplasm (NP-CRN) has a high association with advanced pathology, irrespective of size.[2] Thus, using EMR, a complete pathologic specimen is obtained, the risk of lymph node metastasis can be accurately assessed based on the depth of invasion, and patients can be suitably managed. Used according to its indications, EMR provides curative resection, and obviates the higher morbidity, mortality, and cost associated with surgical treatment.[3,4]

INDICATIONS FOR COLORECTAL EMR

EMR is indicated for the treatment of non-polypoid colorectal lesions when removal at the submucosal level is required to obtain accurate pathology, and ascertain endoscopic cure. For lesions suspected to have high-grade dysplasia or superficial submucosal invasive cancer, EMR is an appropriate strategy and an attempt should be made to remove the lesion en bloc. On the other hand, if piecemeal EMR is technically necessary to remove such lesions with advanced pathology, then the endoscopist should minimize the number of pieces and consider submucosal dissection technique

Veterans Affairs Palo Alto Health Care System, 3801 Miranda Avenue, GI-111, Palo Alto, CA 94304, USA
* Corresponding author.
E-mail address: tonya_kolodziejski@yahoo.com

Gastrointest Endoscopy Clin N Am 20 (2010) 503–514
doi:10.1016/j.giec.2010.03.009
1052-5157/10/$ – see front matter. Published by Elsevier Inc.

or surgical management. EMR is not indicated when the endoscopist does not believe that he or she can remove the entire lesion in one session (**Fig. 1**). EMR can be safe and efficacious but requires knowledge, expertise, time, and a team; without them, EMR can in fact be dangerous (**Fig. 2**). Thus, EMR is not indicated when the endoscopist does not have the expertise to perform it or is not willing to follow the principles of safe practice of EMR. The indications of colonoscopic mucosal resection are shown in **Box 1**.

ESTIMATION OF THE DEPTH OF INVASION

Colonoscopic assessment of the most likely pathology and estimation of the depth of invasion is important in planning an EMR of the colon and rectum. Neoplasm limited to the mucosa is the best target lesion. Lesions with minimal or moderate likelihood to contain submucosal invasion can be treated with EMR for diagnostic and therapeutic purposes, provided that the endoscopist believes that the lesion can be safely removed in its entirety, and that the potential benefits of endoscopic treatment outweigh the risks. Patients whose lesions are strongly suggestive of invasion should be referred to surgery after a confirmatory biopsy, as endoscopic resection will expose them to unnecessary risks. For example, colonoscopic resection of neoplasms with massive submucosal invasive cancer is generally difficult to accomplish and has a high risk of bleeding, perforation, recurrence, and metastasis. It is appropriate, after assessment of the lesion, to reschedule the patient for a dedicated resection procedure. This rescheduling allows appropriate discussion of the risks and

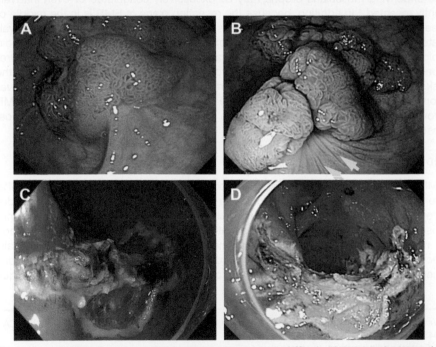

Fig. 1. Repeat EMR of an incomplete prior resection is very difficult. The scar is shown under white light and after indigo carmine spray (*A* and *B*, respectively). The resection was piecemeal as the lesion lift partially (*C*). Such a piecemeal resection produces tissues that are difficult to interpret, thus putting the patient (and physician) at risk. (*D*) The resected site before application of argon plasma coagulation (not shown).

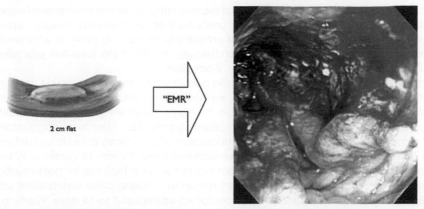

2 cm flat

"EMR"

Fig. 2. Endoscopic mucosal resection of the colon requires multiple detailed steps. The best assessment of pathology requires the EMR specimen to be en bloc and well oriented. In cases where piecemeal resection is performed, it is important to minimize the number of pieces. The picture shows an obstructing lesion of a patient who was referred for an evaluation of constipation. The patient's history recorded a piecemeal EMR performed 2 years earlier at the same location. Reevaluation of the pathology slides showed that the lesion was resected into minute pieces which, in turn, made appropriate pathologic examination impossible.

benefits with the patient, and ensures adequate planning for the necessary equipment, time, and personnel for the procedure.

MANAGEMENT OF ANTICOAGULANT AND ANTIPLATELET MEDICATIONS

In preparation for a *standard* polypectomy colonoscopy procedure, the American Society of Gastrointestinal Endoscopy (ASGE) guidelines recommend no interruption of antiplatelet medications, such as aspirin or nonsteroidal anti-inflammatory drugs, though they do recommend the discontinuation of platelet aggregation inhibitors, such as ticlopidine and clopidogrel, for 7 to 10 days.[5] The ASGE advises that patients on anticoagulation at relatively low risk of thromboembolic complications can discontinue warfarin 5 days before the procedure. The international normalized ratio (INR) should be 1.4 or less, although we (T.K. and R.S., the authors of this article) prefer a normal INR before an EMR. High-risk patients, such as those with atrial fibrillation

---

Box 1
Indications for endoscopic mucosal resection in the colon

1. Without advanced/massive submucosal invasive pathology

2. Any size:

    Lesion requiring resection at the submucosa to ensure cure

    Suspicious high-grade dysplasia/superficial spreading melanoma that can be removed en bloc using the technique

3. Pathology:

    United States: high-grade dysplasia or intramucosal adenocarcinoma

    Japan: well-differentiated adenocarcinoma without lymphovascular involvement up to 1000 μm from the muscularis mucosa

and concomitant valvular disease, should receive either standard intravenous heparin until approximately 6 hours before the procedure or low-molecular-weight heparin until approximately 24 hours before the procedure. Of note, in patients who are on short-term antiplatelet or anticoagulation therapy, we defer the resection procedure until they no longer require such agents, if possible.

In the absence of robust data or specific guidelines for the postresection management of large or complex colon lesions, we typically individualize care for the reinstitution of antiplatelet or anticoagulation therapy, considering both the patient's thromboembolic risk and postresection bleeding potential. After large polypectomy or mucosal resection, we typically use endoscopic clips to close the mucosal defects. We generally instruct patients who have significant risk factors to continue to take aspirin, 81 mg daily. In the rare patient considered to be at high risk for postresection bleeding, we recommend that the patient refrain from taking other nonsteroidal anti-inflammatory drugs, and platelet inhibitors for an additional 7 to 14 days. Warfarin is resumed 10 days after the procedure. In patients at high risk for coagulation, we use intravenous heparin: we resume the heparin infusion 2 to 6 hours after the procedure, until the INR is therapeutic.

In our published experience of colonoscopic resection of small (<1 cm) colorectal lesions in anticoagulated patients, we withheld warfarin for approximately 36 hours only, to avoid supratherapeutic anticoagulation due to dietary restriction and bowel purge. In this retrospective series, using a variety of polypectomy techniques, including cold snare, standard snare with cautery, and inject-and-cut mucosectomy, followed by endoscopic clipping, the risk of major delayed bleeding in the resection of 5.1 ± 2.2 mm lesion was 0.8% (95% confidence interval: 0.1%–4.5%).[6]

MANAGEMENT OF HIGH-RISK PATIENTS FOR BACTERIAL ENDOCARDITIS

We follow the ASGE guidelines. In general, antibiotic prophylaxis is not recommended for EMR. Note, however, that there are limited data for EMR of large colorectal lesion, and exception to the recommendation may be necessary for select patients.

EMR Procedure at Palo Alto

We use a standardized endoscopic resection approach that includes lesion assessment, inject-and-cut EMR (for the colon and rectum), and EMR Ligation (for the rectum only) techniques, immediate reassessment and treatment of residual, histologic preparation and assessment, and surveillance, to safely and efficaciously remove non-polypoid lesions. Note that we do not use other EMR techniques such as the EMR Cap or the Double Channel EMR because of the risks of perforations.

Equipment and Tools

We use therapeutic endoscopes equipped with an auxiliary water jet. We typically use an adult high-definition colonoscope, with the accessory channel at the 5-o'clock position, for right colon lesions or alternatively, a therapeutic gastroscope, with the accessory channel at 7-o'clock, for left-sided lesions. The translucent distal attachment device is often a helpful tool to augment stable visualization and resection, particularly of rectal lesions (**Box 2**).

Assessment

The appearance and border of a non-polypoid lesion is closely examined using white light and image-enhanced endoscopy to assess the histopathology, estimate the depth of invasion, and delineate the neoplastic borders to determine its

---

Box 2
Tools for colonoscopy with endoscopic mucosal resection

1. Colonoscope with auxiliary water jet

2. Diagnostic:

   Adult colonoscope with high-resolution image (minimum)

   Pediatric colonoscope with high-resolution image

3. Therapeutic: adult colonoscope (right sided) or therapeutic upper (left sided)

4. Carbon dioxide regulator

5. Diluted simethicone in 60-mL syringe

6. Indigo carmine in 60-mL syringe

7. Injection needle (diluted indigo carmine in preloaded 10 mL, Spot tattoo)

8. Standard generator (Blend current 35 to 40 W)

9. Stiff snare: 2 types (large and small)

10. Biopsy forceps (cold and hot of standard cup size)

11. Endoscopic clips (naked Resolution, Endoclip). Endoscopic loop. EVL 6 bander

12. Argon plasma coagulator with straight catheter

13. Roth net and multichannel suction trap

---

appropriateness for EMR.[7] Specifically, following the initial lesion inspection with white light, we then examine the mucosal and microvascular pattern of the lesion using NBI (Narrow Band Imaging), FICE (Fuji Intelligent Color Enhancement), or i-Scan, and then spray diluted (0.2%) indigo carmine (American Reagent Laboratories Inc, USA) directly onto the area of the lesion using a syringe through the accessory channel of the endoscope.

DETAILED INJECT-AND-CUT COLORECTAL EMR
"Dynamic" Submucosal Injection

We raise the diseased mucosa away from the muscularis propria by the creation of a submucosal bleb using a saline solution (a mixture of diluted indigo carmine and saline) that is injected with a 25-gauge sclerotherapy needle. The use of indigo carmine in the injectant aids in the rapid visual assessment of resection depth.

In cases of large lesions, we initially inject the periphery of the lesion, typically on the side farthest away from the endoscope tip, before we inject the lateral margins and the periphery of the lesion closest to the endoscope tip. Total injection volume has not been defined and varies according to the size of the lesion; our injection volumes generally range between 10 and 50 mL. We use a dynamic submucosal injection technique (see the article by Soetiknoand and Kaltenbach elsewhere in this issue for further exploration of this topic). We first engage the catheter probe at our intended injection site, expose the needle by instructing our assistant "needle out," then adjust the catheter position further in or out of the accessory channel according to the plane while instructing the assist to "inject." While the assistant is injecting rapidly and steadily, we concomitantly perform dynamic maneuvers to produce a localized submucosal bleb. Specifically, while the submucosal bleb is raised with injection, we slightly adjust the injection catheter position (usually pulling back into the accessory channel), we deflect up with our endoscope tip into the direction of the lumen, and we slightly desufflate the lumen with suction (**Fig. 3**).

Each lesion is closely observed during and after submucosal injection to assess for the nonlifting sign to minimize the risk for a transmural burn or perforation, and assess for submucosal invasion. EMR is performed on any lesion that can be elevated with submucosal injection of fluid. Lifting indicates that there is no deep fixation or only a limited degree of fixation to the submucosal layer, with the probability of complete endoscopic removal. If a complete nonlifting sign is observed then the EMR is aborted, the area is tattooed with injection of carbon black particle solutions (Spot, GI Supply, Camp Hill, PA, USA) and endoscopically clipped, and the patient is referred to surgery. A same-day abdominal radiograph can precisely define the lesion location based on the radio-opaque clip, and can assist in surgical planning.

Snare

We begin our resection where the polyp is easiest to remove. We choose the stiff snare (SD-230U-20, SD-210U-10, Olympus, Center Valley, PA, USA) depending on the lesion size and place it around the lifted area of interest. We keep the lumen insufflated with air for the wall to be stretched to avoid capturing the muscularis propria. However, after we position our snare around the intended lesion, we then slightly suction to collapse the distended colon, and ease snare capturing. Our assistant is

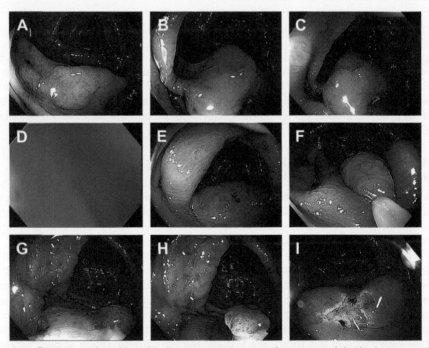

Fig. 3. A flat lesion after diluted indigo carmine image enhancement (*A*). The lesion was injected with saline tinged with indigo carmine. Dynamic submucosal injection was performed (*B* and *C*). During injection, we suctioned the lumen occasionally until a red-out (*D*). Generous submucosal bulge was formed (*E*). The lesion was resected using a stiff snare (*F*). The lesion was lifted away from the wall while the snare was being loosened slightly (*G*) to release any potential entrapment of the muscularis propria. (*H*) The resected lesion. (*I*) The site.

instructed to close the snare until it is "tight" but not transected. In instances when the lesion cannot be captured using this technique, we adjust the approach of the snare to be in a fulcrum position to provide more stiffness during mucosal capture (**Fig. 4**). Once the snare is closed tight, we then re-insufflate air to assess the amount of tissue captured. At this stage, we instruct the assistant to "slightly loosen the snare" and we deflect the endoscopic tip upward. The intent is to release any entrapped muscularis propria, and in fact, if the snare is visible during this "loosening" maneuver, then the assistant has opened the snare too much and there is a risk that the captured lesion will be released out of the snare. Following the proper "loosening" step, we strangulate and resect the lesion with the electrosurgical snare using blended current (30 W right colon, 40 W left colon and rectum using Microvasive Endostat II/III Generator, Boston Scientific, Natick, MA; Endocut using ERBE VIO 300 D Electrosurgical Generator 60 W; ERBE, Atlanta, GA, USA).

Mucosal resection of lesions that are highly suspicious for carcinoma is performed en bloc whenever possible. Such en bloc resection, if possible with surrounding normal mucosa, will provide the ideal specimen for evaluation of involvement of the lateral and vertical margin. To optimize the position, we may even approach the lesion in retroflexed view to achieve en bloc resection (**Fig. 5**). In cases where the lesion cannot be removed by en bloc resection (ie, the entire lesion does not safely fit within the snare), then piecemeal resection is performed.

Reassessment

The completeness of resection is assessed immediately at the time of EMR, and we make every effort to resect each lesion entirely during the initial session. Residual tissue, in fact, may develop underlying fibrosis following electrocoagulation, and thus not lift with subsequent submucosal injection (**Fig. 6**) and ultimately preclude

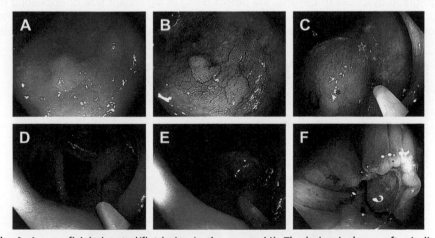

Fig. 4. A superficial elevated/flat lesion in the cecum (A). The lesion is shown after indigo carmine enhancement (B) and submucosal injection (C). The fulcrum technique was used to deploy the snare parallel to the capture the lesion well. The tip of the snare was most optimally positioned at the red arrow. Positioning at the white star would have caused the snare to slip, whereas positioning at the black asterisk would cause an incomplete resection. The fulcrum technique requires the assistant to open the snare slowly while the endoscopist moves the tip of the endoscope to the left (D), keeping the tip of the snare secure and the width of the snare to capture the entire lesion. (E) The lesion had been captured. (F) The resected site after en bloc resection.

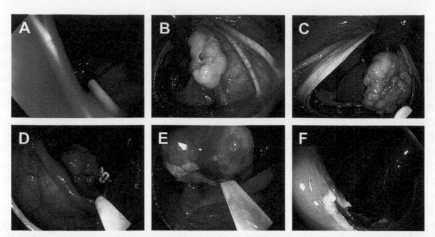

Fig. 5. Endoscopic resection is useful in the resection of large sessile lesions; in this case a sessile lesion behind a fold in the hepatic flexure. The lesion was barely visible (*A*). Submucosal injection would have been difficult. The lesion was better seen on retroflexion (*B*) allowing dynamic submucosal resection to be performed (*C*). The snare was being opened (*D*) and tightened (*E*), capturing the lesion in one piece. (*F*) The resected site.

repeat resection. Thus, in our practice, we complete inject-and-cut EMR at the time of the initial resection to remove any area of visible residual tissue. We then apply argon plasma coagulation using forced mode settings at 1.2 L/min gas flow and 60 W to the periphery of the EMR sites, as well as to exposed vessels (**Fig. 7**). Endoscopic clipping to approximate the mucosal defect may be performed in cases unlikely to be high-grade dysplasia or beyond, the defect being of significant size or appearing to touch the muscularis propria. Other considerations include the lesion being in the cecum or ascending colon and the patient coming from a remote location. Note

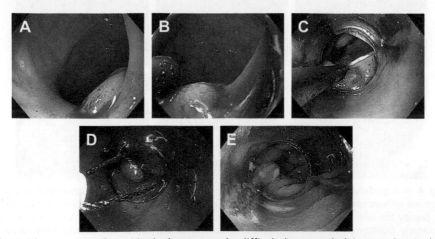

Fig. 6. The resection of a residual adenoma can be difficult due to underlying scarring. In this case, the residual lesion was also behind a fold and a sigmoid turn (*A*). The use of the appropriate cap is important as it can provide a mechanism to remove the lesion completely. The lesion was unable to be visualized using a short cap (*B*). The lesion was fully seen using a banding cap, allowing submucosal injection (*C*) and snaring (*D*). (*E*) The resection site.

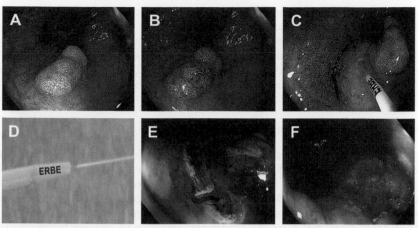

Fig. 7. A sessile lesion in the rectum under white light (*A*) and narrow-band imaging (*B*). The submucosa was injected using the ERBE Lift (*C*), a needleless injector system that provides a fast and thin jet of saline (*D*). In our unit, after EMR we would ablate the visible capillaries and venules using argon plasma coagulation (*E* and *F*). Larger vessels usually require clip applications (not shown).

that there is a limited literature on the routine use of clipping post EMR to close a mucosal defect.

Following endoscopic treatment, we inject carbon black submucosally to mark lesions larger than 2 cm and those suspicious of harboring invasive carcinoma.

Specimen Retrieval and Preparation

A snare net (Roth net, US Endoscopy, Mentor, OH, USA) is used to retrieve the intact resected specimen for histologic processing to prevent fragmentation of the specimen. We stretch and fix the retrieved specimen using fine pins inserted at the periphery of the lesion into a plate of Styrofoam or wood to orient the specimen before pathologic fixation, and to prevent retraction and curling of the tissue. Fixed specimens are sectioned serially at 2-mm intervals parallel to a line that includes the closest resection margin of the specimen. This preparation and sectioning technique allows careful analysis of the histologic type, degree of differentiation, depth of vertical invasion, presence of ulceration, vessel involvement, and invasion of cancer into the resected margins. The resection can be diagnosed as complete or incomplete–complete when both the horizontal and vertical margins are negative. Lesions that are resected piecemeal with EMR cannot be precisely reconfigured and may be too small to pin out, and thus can be difficult to stage accurately.

Surveillance Colonoscopy

An EMR resection is considered complete when the endoscopic margins are macroscopically disease free and both the horizontal and vertical cauterized histopathologic margins are free of neoplasm. We perform surveillance colonoscopy at 3 to 6 months to assess for local recurrence in patients who underwent piecemeal resection. We refer patients with submucosal invasive carcinoma or lesions not amenable to curative EMR for surgical resection.

On surveillance colonoscopy, we locate the prior EMR site based on a scar or tattoo. We inspect the innominate groove pattern closely to macroscopically assess for local recurrence using both high-definition, electronic-based image-enhanced endoscopy and diluted indigo carmine (0.2%). Repeat EMR is performed for local recurrence (**Fig. 8**). Biopsies are obtained of the scarred site of lesions with advanced pathology if there is no macroscopic evidence of recurrence. In general, after a clearing examination we repeat the examination at 1 and 3 years, although patients with giant lesions may undergo three successive yearly examinations.

CLINICAL OUTCOMES OF EMR

Numerous studies have shown that large colorectal lesions can be safely and effectively removed endoscopically.[8–14] The current data primarily reflect the resection outcomes of both sessile and non-polypoid lesions by expert endoscopists. However, long-term efficacy and cost data on EMR of large non-polypoid (flat and depressed) colorectal lesions is limited. As such, the majority of non-polypoid lesions are typically referred for surgery due a variety of reasons including insufficient technical skills, perceived high complication risk, increased use of endoscopy resources and time, and inadequate reimbursement.[15,16]

Preliminary data from our referral cohort of 240 non-polypoid lesions with a mean size of 24.5 ± 12.0 mm (range 10–80 mm) showed a low surgical referral rate of 13.3%. Specifically, we obviated the need for surgery in 86.7% of the patients by successful endoscopic removal of non-polypoid colorectal lesions. These were non-polypoid lesions referred by gastroenterologists (n = 189) and surgeons (n = 51); a third (n = 80) of them had previous incomplete endoscopic treatment. In fact, our main reason for surgical referral was nonlifting sign (n = 20), followed by invasive pathology (n = 8), involvement of the appendiceal orifice (n = 2), or large precluding safe resection (n = 2). Post-EMR surveillance data in close to half of the patients

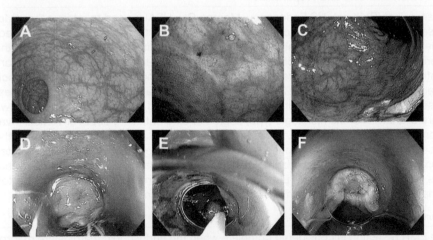

Fig. 8. This patient was referred for evaluation of an EMR site, which on prior biopsy showed villous adenoma. The site of recurrence was difficult to visualize. With high-definition endoscopy, the site was visible as a reddish area with adenomatous mucosal pattern (*A*). Indigo carmine chromoscopy was used, but did not add additional information (*B*). The site was marked using small bursts of cautery that were applied using the tip of a snare (*C*). EMR using ligation, which is used only in the rectum, was used. (*D*) The recurrence site before band ligation, and (*E*) while it was being snared under the band. (*F*) The resection site. The pathology revealed villous adenoma with surrounding normal mucosa (not shown).

showed 14.9% (n = 17/114) local recurrence rate with a mean size of 4.5 ± 2.7 mm (range 1–10 mm) that were successfully treated endoscopically.

In our longer term efficacy study of standardized inject-and-cut EMR technique on 125 non-polypoid lesions (117 flat and 8 depressed) with a mean size of 16.7 ± 7 mm (range 10–50 mm), we found a 10% rate of local recurrence at the prior EMR site at the first surveillance colonoscopy, with ultimate eradication following 1 or 2 additional colonoscopies.[17] Of note, the recurrence was small (mean size 4 mm). No lesion required surgery. Over a 4.5-year follow up period, no patient developed or died of advanced colorectal cancer or distant metastasis.

Others have published recurrence rates of more than 40% following piecemeal endoscopic resection of large colorectal lesions.[18,19] Local recurrence does not equate to endoscopic treatment failure, but rather it should remind us of the importance of intensive postresection surveillance and retreatment. A recent series of approximately 300 polyps larger than 3 cm that were resected endoscopically demonstrated a recurrence rate of 17%, with the majority of recurrent lesions successfully treated endoscopically.[20] In cases with residual neoplasia, appropriate therapy with biopsy or repeat EMR is prudent, and another surveillance colonoscopy should be performed at 6 months. Subsequent examinations should be performed at 3 to 6 months until long-term eradication is confirmed, and then the patient should resume surveillance at the recommended guideline intervals. Khashab and colleagues[21,22] reported a high predictive value for long-term eradication in cases where the postmucosectomy scar site showed both normal macroscopic and microscopic (biopsy) findings.

COMPLICATIONS OF EMR

Despite general perceptions of high complication rates associated with EMR, skilled endoscopists have reported low adverse events. In comparison to the 20.1% morbidity and 1.3% mortality rates for laparoscopic or open surgery of colon tumors, general EMR data show rates of 0.7% to 3.7% for perforation and 0.4% to 3.8% for bleeding.[23] The risks of EMR, however, can be further decreased. Based on our cumulative EMR data, we inform patients of a 1 in 250 chance of postresection bleeding that can be treated with endoscopic hemostasis, and a theoretical risk of perforation.

SUMMARY

EMR using the inject-and-cut technique is a safe and efficacious approach for large flat neoplasms, high-grade dysplasia, or mucosal carcinomas in the colon and rectum.

REFERENCES

1. Soetikno RM, Gotoda T, Nakanishi Y, et al. Endoscopic mucosal resection. Gastrointest Endosc 2003;57:567–79.
2. Soetikno RM, Kaltenbach T, Rouse RV, et al. Prevalence of nonpolypoid (flat and depressed) colorectal neoplasms in asymptomatic and symptomatic adults. JAMA 2008;299:1027–35.
3. Soetikno R, Kaltenbach T, Yeh R, et al. Endoscopic mucosal resection for early cancers of the upper gastrointestinal tract. J Clin Oncol 2005;23:4490–8.
4. Soetikno R, Gotoda T. Con: colonoscopic resection of large neoplastic lesions is appropriate and safe. Am J Gastroenterol 2009;104:272–5.
5. Anderson MA, Ben-Menachem T, Gan SI, et al. Management of antithrombotic agents for endoscopic procedures. Gastrointest Endosc 2009;70:1060–70.

6. Friedland S, Sedehi D, Soetikno R. Colonoscopic polypectomy in anticoagulated patients. World J Gastroenterol 2009;15:1973–6.

7. Soetikno RM, Fujii T, Friedland S, et al. Diagnosis of flat and depressed colorectal neoplasms - An educational DVD. ASGE Learning Center. Chicago: American Society Gastrointestinal Endoscopy; 2004.

8. Kanamori T, Itoh M, Yokoyama Y, et al. Injection-incision-assisted snare resection of large sessile colorectal polyp. Gastrointest Endosc 1996;43:189–95.

9. Tanaka S, Haruma K, Oka S, et al. Clinicopathologic features and endoscopic treatment of superficially spreading colorectal neoplasms larger than 20 mm. Gastrointest Endosc 2001;54:62–6.

10. Su MY, Hsu CM, Ho YP, et al. Endoscopic mucosal resection for colonic non-polypoid neoplasms. Am J Gastroenterol 2005;100:2174–9.

11. Bergmann U, Beger HG. Endoscopic mucosal resection for advanced non-polypoid colorectal adenoma and early stage carcinoma. Surg Endosc 2003; 17:475–9.

12. Arebi N, Swain D, Suzuki N, et al. Endoscopic mucosal resection of 161 cases of large sessile or flat colorectal polyps. Scand J Gastroenterol 2007;42:859–66.

13. Luigiano C, Consolo P, Scaffidi MG, et al. Endoscopic mucosal resection for large and giant sessile and flat colorectal polyps: a single-center experience with long-term follow-up. Endoscopy 2009;41:829–35.

14. Regula J, Wronska E, Polkowski M, et al. Argon plasma coagulation after piece-meal polypectomy of sessile colorectal adenomas: long-term follow-up study. Endoscopy 2003;35:212–8.

15. Overhiser AJ, Rex DK. Work and resources needed for endoscopic resection of large sessile colorectal polyps. Clin Gastroenterol Hepatol 2007;5:1076–9.

16. Swan MP, Bourke MJ, Alexander S, et al. Large refractory colonic polyps: is it time to change our practice? A prospective study of the clinical and economic impact of a tertiary referral colonic mucosal resection and polypectomy service (with videos). Gastrointest Endosc 2009;70:1128–36.

17. Kaltenbach T, Friedland S, Maheshwari A, et al. Short- and long-term outcomes of standardized EMR of nonpolypoid (flat and depressed) colorectal lesions > or = 1 cm (with video). Gastrointest Endosc 2007;65:857–65.

18. Brooker JC, Saunders BP, Shah SG, et al. Treatment with argon plasma coagulation reduces recurrence after piecemeal resection of large sessile colonic polyps: a randomized trial and recommendations. Gastrointest Endosc 2002;55:371–5.

19. Iishi H, Tatsuta M, Iseki K, et al. Endoscopic piecemeal resection with submucosal saline injection of large sessile colorectal polyps. Gastrointest Endosc 2000;51:697–700.

20. Seitz U, Bohnacker S, Seewald S, et al. Long-term results of endoscopic removal of large colorectal adenomas. Endoscopy 2003;35:S41–4.

21. Khashab M, Eid E, Rusche M, et al. Incidence and predictors of "late" recurrences after endoscopic piecemeal resection of large sessile adenomas. Gastrointest Endosc 2009;70:344–9.

22. Rose J, Schneider C, Yildirim C, et al. Complications in laparoscopic colorectal surgery: results of a multicentre trial. Tech Coloproctol 2004;8(Suppl 1):s25–8.

23. The Clinical Outcomes of Surgical Therapy Study Group. A comparison of laparoscopically assisted and open colectomy for colon cancer. N Engl J Med 2004; 350:2050–9.

Endoscopic Submucosal Dissection of Non-Polypoid Colorectal Neoplasms

Yutaka Saito, MD, PhD[a],*, Takahisa Matsuda, MD, PhD[a],
Takahiro Fujii, MD, PhD[b]

KEYWORDS

- Endoscopic submucosal dissection
- Endoscopic mucosal resection
- Endoscopic piecemeal mucosal resection • Colorectum
- Laterally spreading tumor granular type
- Laterally spreading tumor nongranular type

Traditionally, endoscopic mucosal resection (EMR)[1–5] and surgery were the only available treatments for large colorectal tumors, even for those detected at an early stage. In Japan, EMR is indicated for the treatment of colorectal adenomas, intramucosal and submucosal superficial (invasion <1000 μm from the muscularis mucosae) cancers, because of its negligible risk of lymph node metastasis[6] and excellent clinical outcomes.[2–4]

The endoscopic submucosal dissection (ESD) technique, which enables en-bloc resection of large tumors, is accepted as a standard minimally invasive treatment for early gastric cancer in Japan.[7,8] However, it is not widely used to treat superficial colorectal cancer because of technical difficulty and the higher risk of complications. Conventional EMR, therefore, is used for the resection of non-polypoid colorectal neoplasms (NP-CRNs), including the large flat carpet lesions, called colorectal laterally spreading tumors (LSTs).[4,5] EMR, however, is not designed for en-bloc resection of LSTs larger than 20 mm. Piecemeal EMR is associated with the risks of incomplete removal and local recurrence[9] albeit most recurrences can be successfully treated by additional EMR and only a few cases require surgery.[9] ESD of LSTs larger than 20 mm is therefore an attractive treatment provided that it is safe to use in the colon and rectum.

[a] Endoscopy Division, National Cancer Center Hospital, 5-1-1 Tsukiji, Chuo-ku, Tokyo 104-0045, Japan
[b] Fujii Takahiro Clinic, Chuo-ku, Tokyo, Japan
* Corresponding author.
E-mail address: ytsaito@ncc.go.jp

Gastrointest Endoscopy Clin N Am 20 (2010) 515–524
doi:10.1016/j.giec.2010.03.010
1052-5157/10/$ – see front matter © 2010 Elsevier Inc. All rights reserved.

Based on the refinement of ESD instruments and progress in the development of ESD skills, the ESD technique has recently been reported to be useful in the treatment of large colorectal LSTs instead of EMR or surgery.[10–15] Herein, the authors describe their experience.

INDICATIONS FOR COLORECTAL ESD

The indication for colorectal ESD at the National Cancer Center Hospital (NCCH) in Tokyo, Japan, is a nongranular type LST (LST-NG) larger than 20 mm.[12]

Based on clinicopathologic analyses of LSTs,[4,16] LST-NGs, which are large (>1 cm) superficial elevated NP-CRNs with a smooth surface, have a higher rate of submucosal (sm) invasion, which can be difficult to predict endoscopically. About 30% of LST-NGs with sm invasions are multifocal, and such invasions are primarily superficial submucosal cancers (sm1s) and difficult to predict before endoscopic treatment.

Granular type LSTs (LST-Gs) have a lower rate of sm invasion, and most such invasions are found under the largest nodule or depression, which are easier to predict endoscopically.[4,16] LST-Gs larger than 20 mm can be treated by endoscopic piecemeal mucosal resection (EPMR) rather than by ESD, with the area that has the largest nodule resected before resection of the remaining tumor. LST-Gs larger than 30 mm or 40 mm are possible candidates for ESD because they have higher sm invasion rates and are more difficult to treat even by EPMR; so they have been treated by either EPMR or ESD, based on the individual endoscopist's judgment.

ESTIMATION OF THE DEPTH OF INVASION

A non-invasive pattern[17,18] should be verified in each lesion, indicating suitability for EMR or ESD: the estimated invasion depth should be less than that of superficial submucosal cancers (sm1s). No biopsy is performed before ESD because it can cause fibrosis and may interfere with submucosal lifting.

CESSATION PERIOD OF ANTICOAGULANT AND ANTIPLATELET BEFORE ESD

ESD is considered to be a high-risk procedure.[19] Most patients receiving aspirin or ticlopidine alone underwent ESD after a cessation period of 5 to 7 days and restarted the drugs after 7 days if possible. Patients receiving warfarin used intravenous heparin or subcutaneous low-molecular-weight heparin in the perioperative period and resumed warfarin after the ESD procedure.

ESD PROCEDURE AT NCCH

The procedures were primarily performed using a ball-tip bipolar needle knife (B-knife) (XEMEX Co, Tokyo Japan) (**Fig. 1**A)[20] and an insulation-tip (IT) electrosurgical knife (Olympus Optical Co, Tokyo, Japan) (see **Fig. 1**B) with carbon dioxide insufflations instead of air insufflation to reduce patient discomfort (see **Fig. 1**C).[11] After submucosal injection of 10% glycerin and 5% fructose (Glyceol, Chugai Pharmaceutical Co, Tokyo, Japan)[21] and 0.4% hyaluronic acid[14] (MucoUp, Seikakagu Co, Tokyo, Japan) (see **Fig. 1**D) into the sm layer, a circumferential incision was made using the B-knife and an ESD was then performed using the B-knife and IT knife (see **Fig. 1**A, B).

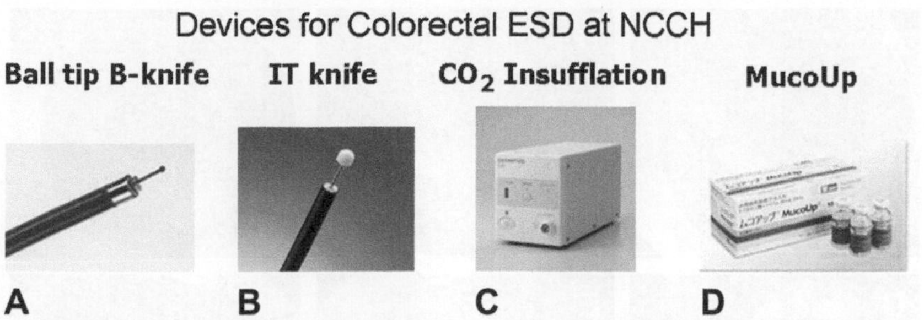

Devices for Colorectal ESD at NCCH

Ball tip B-knife   **IT knife**   **CO$_2$ Insufflation**   **MucoUp**

A   B   C   D

Fig. 1. The procedures were primarily performed using a B-knife (A) and an IT electrosurgical knife (B) with carbon dioxide insufflation (C) instead of air insufflation to reduce patient discomfort. After injection of Glyceol (Chugai Pharmaceutical Co, Tokyo, Japan) and MucoUp (Seikakagu Co, Tokyo, Japan) (D) into the sm layer, a circumferential incision was made using the B-knife and an ESD was performed using the B-knife and IT knife. (*From* XEMEX Co, Tokyo, Japan; with permission [A]; Olympus Optical Co, Tokyo, Japan; with permission [B]; and Seikakagu Co, Tokyo, Japan; with permission [D].)

SUBMUCOSAL INJECTION SOLUTION

A mixture of 2 solutions was prepared before the procedure to create a longer-lasting sm fluid cushion.

Solution 1: Indigo carmine dye (2 mL of 1% solution) and epinephrine (1 mL of 0.1% solution) were mixed with 200 mL Glyceol[21] in a container, which was then drawn into a 5-mL disposable syringe.

Solution 2: MucoUp was drawn into another 5-mL syringe with a smaller amount of indigo carmine dye and epinephrine. During the actual ESD procedure, a small amount of solution 1 was injected into the sm layer to confirm the appropriate sm layer elevation and then solution 2 was injected into the properly elevated sm layer. Finally, a small amount of solution 1 was injected again to flush out any residual solution 2.

DETAILED COLORECTAL ESD PROCEDURES

1. The margins of the lesion were delineated before ESD by spraying 0.4% indigo carmine dye (**Fig. 2**A). After creation of the submucosal fluid cushion, an initial incision was made with the B-knife at the oral side of the lesion (see **Fig. 2**B).[20] In colorectal cases, it was not necessary to actually mark around lesions because tumor margins can be visualized clearly with indigo carmine.

2. The B-knife was inserted into the initial incision, and an electrosurgical current was applied in endocut mode (50 W) using a standard electrosurgical generator (ICC 200, ERBE, Tubingen, Germany) to continue the marginal incision around the oral side of the lesion.

3. After partial resection of the margin on the oral side of the lesion to ensure adequate submucosal lifting, submucosal dissection was begun using the same B-knife in retroflex view (see **Fig. 2**B).

4. Additional resection of the margin on the anal side was performed using the B-knife in the straight view (see **Fig. 2**C).

5. After the lesion was partially dissected so that the sm layer could be visualized sufficiently, an IT knife (see **Fig. 2**D) was used to complete the dissection of the sm layer quickly and safely. The previously indicated solutions were injected

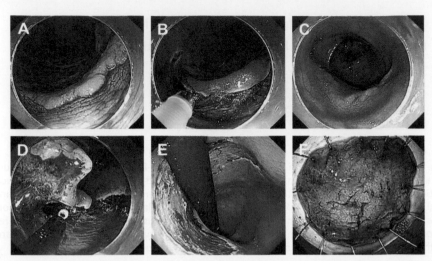

Fig. 2. ESD procedures. (*A*) An LST-NG type lesion 40 mm in size located in transverse colon (reverse view). Lesion margins delineated before ESD using 0.4% indigo carmine dye spraying. (*B*) After injection of Glyceol and sodium hyaluronate acid solution into the sm layer, a half-circumferential incision (anal side) was performed using B-knife (retroflex view). After circumferential incision, sm dissection was performed using the same B-knife. (*C*) Straight view of the lesion after half-circumference marginal resection and sm dissection of the oral side. Additional resection of the margin on the anal side was performed using the B-knife in the straight view. (*D*) Dissection of the sm layer from outside to inside of the lesion is easily performed using the IT knife. (*E*) Ulcer bed after successful en-bloc resection in 1.5 hours. (*F*) Resected specimen was 40 × 30 mm in diameter and histologic findings revealed intramucosal cancer with tumor-free margin.

   repeatedly into the sm layer to maintain the sm fluid cushion so as to minimize the risk of perforation.
6. Hemostatic forceps were used in soft coagulation mode (70–80 W) to control visible bleeding. The patient's position was sometimes changed to facilitate visualization of the tissue plane, and dissection continued until the lesion was completely excised.
7. After the colorectal ESD was completed, routine colonoscopic review to detect any possible perforation or exposed vessels was conducted and minimum coagulation was performed using hemostatic forceps on nonbleeding visible vessels to prevent postoperative bleeding (see **Fig. 2**E).
8. The resected specimen was stretched and fixed to the board using small pins (see **Fig. 2**F).

CLINICAL OUTCOME OF ESD AT NCCH

The en-bloc resection rate was 88% and the curative resection rate was 86% among 500 ESDs (**Table 1**). Of these, 127 were tubular adenomas, 315 were intramucosal cancers or minute sm cancers (sm1s), 55 were submucosal deep cancers (sm2s), 2 were carcinoid tumors, and 1 was mucosa-associated lymphoma tissue. The median operation time was 90 minutes, and the mean size of resected specimens was 40 mm (range, 20–150 mm).

COMPLICATIONS OF ESD AT NCCH

The postoperative bleeding rate for ESD was 1.0% (5 of 500), which is almost the same as that for conventional EMR (see **Table 1**). In contrast, the perforation rate for ESD

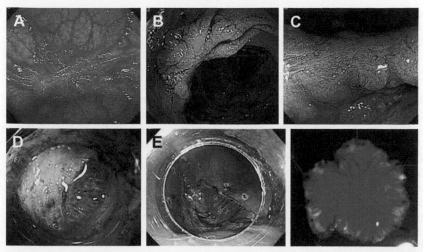

Fig. 3. ESD procedures for recurrent tumor. (*A*) A 20-mm flat-type lesion with ulcer scar was located in the transverse colon, and prominent fold convergences were noticed. (*B*) Lesion margins were delineated before ESD using 0.4% indigo carmine dye spraying. (*C*) Crystal violet (0.05%) staining clearly revealed IIIL and IIIs (non-invasive) pit pattern and indicated that this lesion was a good candidate for endoscopic treatment despite severe fibrosis and nonlifting sign. (*D*) After injection of Glyceol and sodium hyaluronate acid solution into the sm layer, circumferential incision was performed using B-knife. After circumferential incision, sm dissection was performed using B-knife and IT knife. Severe sm layer fibrosis was visualized clearly due to the distal attachment, and the sm layer was carefully dissected just below this fibrosis. (*E*) Ulcer bed after successful en-bloc resection in 1 hour. (*F*) Resected specimen was 20 mm in diameter, and histologic findings revealed intramucosal cancer with tumor-free margin.

Table 1	
Clinical outcomes of 500 colorectal ESDs at NCCH	
Macroscopic Types	
LST-G/LST-NG	220/200
Depressed/Protruded	18/30
Recurrence	28
SMT	4
Location	C:35, Rt: 195, Lt: 130, R:140
Size of Resected Specimens [Mean±SD (range)]	40 ± 20 (20–150) mm
Pathology	Adenoma, 127; m-sm1, 315; sm2, approximately 55; Others, 3
Procedure Time	90 ± 73 (15–390) min
En-bloc Resection	88%
Curative Resection	86%
Complications	
Perforation	13[a] (2.6%)
Delayed Bleeding	5 (1%)

Abbreviations: C, cecum; Lt, left; m-sm1, intramucosal-submucosal superficial (invasive <1000 mm from the muscularis mucosae) cancer; R, rectum; Rt, right; sm2, submucosal deep; SD, standard deviation; SMT, submucosal tumor.
[a] All cases except 1 treated without surgery.

was 2.6% (13 of 500), which is considerably higher than that for conventional EMR (1.3%); only 1 perforation case needed emergency surgery because of ineffective endoscopic clipping. There have been no delayed perforations observed.

TECHNICAL PROGRESS OF COLORECTAL ESD

Until recently, colorectal ESDs have been performed mainly in Japan[10–15,22,23] because of the technical difficulty involved in the procedure. Also, the most frequent indication for ESD, early gastric cancer, is more common in Japan than in Western countries.[24] Some trained endoscopists, however, have started to do colorectal ESDs in Europe[25] and the United States.[26]

Given the thinness of the colonic wall, the use of specialized knives,[7,20] distal attachments,[14] and hypertonic solutions (Glycerol[21] and MucoUp[14]) that produce a longer-lasting and higher sm elevation cushion are necessary for safe ESD and to reduce the perforation rate. The B-knife[20] is safer because the electric current is limited to the needle and the bipolar system prevents electric current from passing to the muscle layer.

A noninvasive and simple tool that facilitates the direct visualization of the sm layer was needed to reduce the risk of perforations in colorectal ESD. As a result, the authors developed a sinker system for traction-assisted ESD[10] and more recently a thin-endoscope–assisted ESD.[27] In addition, Sakamoto and colleagues[28] reported the usefulness of a new traction device (S-O clip) for ESD of superficial colorectal neoplasms.

ESD enables us to treat recurrent lesions after incomplete endoscopic resections (see **Fig. 3; Fig. 4**) and large colorectal LSTs greater than 10 cm in diameter (**Fig. 5**). It is important, therefore, to diagnose the lesion carefully using chromomagnification colonoscopy[17,18] before treatment to reduce unnecessary noncurative resection for sm deep invasive cancers.[6]

COMPARISON BETWEEN ESD AND EMR

The primary advantage of ESD compared with EPMR is a higher en-bloc resection rate for large colonic tumors that had been treated by surgery previously. Consequently, ESD has a lower recurrence rate compared with EPMR (2% vs 14%) and also results

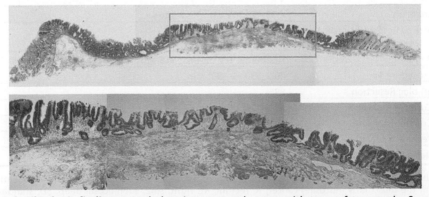

Fig. 4. Histologic findings revealed an intramucosal cancer with tumor-free margin. Severe fibrosis caused by previous EMR was observed at the center of this lesion.

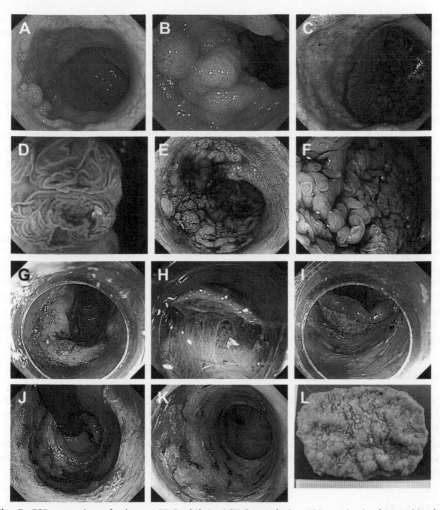

Fig. 5. ESD procedures for large LST-Gs. (*A*) An LST-G type lesion 100 mm in size located in the sigmoid colon. (*B*) A large nodule was identified in this LST-G. (*C*) Narrow-band imaging (NBI) revealed this LST-G lesion as brownish and the margin of this lesion became apparent. (*D*) NBI with magnification revealed a type II or IIIA Sano capillary pattern, suggesting intramucosal neoplastic lesion. (*E*) Lesion margins were delineated before ESD using 0.4% indigo carmine dye spraying. (*F*) Magnification colonoscopy with indigo carmine dye revealed non-invasive (IV) pit pattern at the elevated area of this lesion. (*G*) After injection of Glyceol and sodium hyaluronate acid solution into the sm layer, half-circumferential incision was performed using B-knife. (*H*) and (*I*) After circumferential incision, sm dissection was performed using B-knife and IT knife. Thickened sm layer was visualized as blue because of the distal attachment and indigo carmine. Sm dissection was performed carefully at this thickened sm layer above the muscle layer. (*J*) and (*K*) Ulcer bed after successful en-bloc resection in 2 hours. (*L*) Resected specimen was 100 mm in diameter, and histologic findings revealed intramucosal cancer with tumor-free margin.

in a better quality of life for patients compared with surgery. Future studies should be designed to compare the clinical outcomes of ESD and surgery but not of ESD and EMR because the indications for ESD and EMR are different as are the tumor characteristics.

Until now, EPMR had been considered a feasible treatment for colorectal LSTs. Low rates of local recurrence for such tumors and of repeat endoscopic resection were considered sufficient for most local recurrent tumors.[9]

In the authors' case series,[29] EPMR was also effective in treating many LST-Gs 20 mm or larger, but 3 cases (1.3%) required surgery after such piecemeal resections, including 2 cases of invasive recurrence.

Based on these results, cases for EPMRs in which accurate histologic evaluation would be difficult to make should be considered for ESD or laparoscopic surgery.

LST-Gs larger than 30 mm are good candidates for ESD. The sm invasion rate for such lesions was 16%, and multifocal invasion rate outside the large nodule or depression was 25%, which was more difficult to diagnose even using magnification colonoscopy.

INSTRUCTIONS ON POST-ESD CARE

From data analysis between ESD and EMR, follow-up endoscopy is recommended after 1 year for curative en-bloc ESD cases and after 6 months for piecemeal ESD cases considering local recurrence rates.[28] Even for pathologic curative resection cases, computed tomographic examination or endoscopic ultrasound imaging is recommended to examine lymph node metastasis or distant metastasis for sm1 cases and piecemeal resection cases.

Surgery is recommended for sm2s or cancers of deeper invasion or when lymphovascular invasion is diagnosed histologically.[6]

SUMMARY

ESD is a safe and effective procedure for treating colorectal LST-NGs larger than 20 mm and LST-Gs larger than 30 mm because it has a higher en-bloc resection rate and is less invasive than surgery. Establishment of a training system for technically more difficult colorectal ESD and further refinement of ESD instruments are encouraged for the increased use of colorectal ESD not only in Japan but also throughout the world.

REFERENCES

1. Ahmad NA, Kochman ML, Long WB, et al. Efficacy, safety, and clinical outcomes of endoscopic mucosal resection: a study of 101 cases. Gastrointest Endosc 2002;55:390–6.
2. Yokota T, Sugihara K, Yoshida S. Endoscopic mucosal resection for colorectal neoplastic lesions. Dis Colon Rectum 1994;37:1108–11.
3. Soetikno RM, Gotoda T, Nakanishi Y, et al. Endoscopic mucosal resection. Gastrointest Endosc 2003;57(4):567–79.
4. Saito Y, Fujii T, Kondo H, et al. Endoscopic treatment for laterally spreading tumors in the colon. Endoscopy 2001;33:682–6.
5. Kudo S, Kashida H, Tamura T, et al. Colonoscopic diagnosis and management of nonpolypoid early colorectal cancer. World J Surg 2000;24:1081–90.
6. Kitajima K, Fujimori T, Fujii S, et al. Correlations between lymph node metastasis and depth of submucosal invasion in submucosal invasive colorectal carcinoma: a Japanese collaborative study. J Gastroenterol 2004;39(6):534–43.
7. Hosokawa K, Yoshida S. [Recent advances in endoscopic mucosal resection for early gastric cancer]. Gan To Kagaku Ryoho 1998;25:476–83 [in Japanese].

8. Ono H, Kondo H, Gotoda T, et al. Endoscopic mucosal resection for treatment of early gastric cancer. Gut 2001;48:225–9.
9. Hotta K, Fujii T, Saito Y, et al. Local recurrence after endoscopic resection of colorectal tumors. Int J Colorectal Dis 2009;24(2):225–30.
10. Saito Y, Emura F, Matsuda T, et al. A new sinker-assisted endoscopic submucosal dissection for colorectal tumors. Gastrointest Endosc 2005;62:297–301.
11. Saito Y, Uraoka T, Matsuda T, et al. A pilot study to assess safety and efficacy of carbon dioxide insufflation during colorectal endoscopic submucosal dissection under conscious sedation. Gastrointest Endosc 2007;65(3):537–42.
12. Saito Y, Uraoka T, Matsuda T, et al. Endoscopic treatment of large superficial colorectal tumors: a cases series of 200 endoscopic submucosal dissections (with video). Gastrointest Endosc 2007;66(5):966–73.
13. Yamazaki K, Saito Y, Fukuzawa M. Endoscopic submucosal dissection of a large laterally spreading tumor in the rectum is a minimally invasive treatment. Clin Gastroenterol Hepatol 2008;6(1):e5–6.
14. Yamamoto H, Kawata H, Sunada K, et al. Successful en-bloc resection of large superficial tumors in the stomach and colon using sodium hyaluronate and small-caliber-tip transparent hood. Endoscopy 2003;35:690–4.
15. Fujishiro M, Yahagi N, Kakushima N, et al. Outcomes of endoscopic submucosal dissection for colorectal epithelial neoplasms in 200 consecutive cases. Clin Gastroenterol Hepatol 2007;5(6):674–7.
16. Uraoka T, Saito Y, Matsuda T, et al. Endoscopic indications for endoscopic mucosal resection of laterally spreading tumours in the colorectum. Gut 2006; 55(11):1592–7.
17. Fujii T, Hasegawa RT, Saitoh Y, et al. Chromoscopy during colonoscopy. Endoscopy 2001;33:1036–41.
18. Matsuda T, Fujii T, Saito Y, et al. Efficacy of the invasive/non-invasive pattern by magnifying estimate the depth of invasion of early colorectal neoplasms. Am J Gastroenterol 2008;103(11):2700–6.
19. Friedland S, Sedehi D, Soetikno R. Colonoscopic polypectomy in anticoagulated patients. World J Gastroenterol 2009;15(16):1973–6.
20. Sano Y, Fu KI, Saito Y, et al. A newly developed bipolar-current needle-knife for endoscopic submucosal dissection of large colorectal tumors. Endoscopy 2006;38(Suppl 5):E95.
21. Uraoka T, Fujii T, Saito Y, et al. Effectiveness of glycerol as a submucosal injection for EMR. Gastrointest Endosc 2005;61(6):736–40.
22. Tamegai Y, Saito Y, Masaki N, et al. Endoscopic submucosal dissection: a safe technique for colorectal tumors. Endoscopy 2007;39:418–22.
23. Tanaka S, Oka S, Kaneko I, et al. Endoscopic submucosal dissection for colorectal neoplasia: possibility of standardization. Gastrointest Endosc 2007;66(1): 100–7.
24. Soetikno R, Kaltenbach T, Yeh R, et al. Endoscopic mucosal resection for early cancers of the upper gastrointestinal tract [review]. J Clin Oncol 2005;23(20): 4490–8.
25. Hurlstone DP, Atkinson R, Sanders DS, et al. Achieving R0 resection in the colorectum using endoscopic submucosal dissection. Br J Surg 2007;94(12): 1536–42.
26. Antillon MR, Bartalos CR, Miller ML, et al. En bloc endoscopic submucosal dissection of a 14-cm laterally spreading adenoma of the rectum with involvement to the anal canal: expanding the frontiers of endoscopic surgery (with video). Gastrointest Endosc 2008;67(2):332–7.

27. Uraoka T, Kato J, Ishikawa S, et al. Thin endoscope-assisted endoscopic submucosal dissection for large colorectal tumors (with videos). Gastrointest Endosc 2007;66:836–9.
28. Sakamoto N, Osada T, Shibuya T, et al. The facilitation of a new traction device (S-O clip) assisting endoscopic submucosal dissection for superficial colorectal neoplasms. Endoscopy 2008;40(S 02):E94–5.
29. Saito Y, Fukuzawa M, Matsuda T, et al. Clinical outcome of endoscopic submucosal dissection versus endoscopic mucosal resection of large colorectal tumors as determined by curative resection. Surg Endosc 2010;24(2):343–52.

Non-Polypoid Colorectal Neoplasms in Ulcerative Colitis

Yoshitaka Ueno, MD, PhD[a],*, Shinji Tanaka, MD, PhD[a],
Kazuaki Chayama, MD, PhD[b]

KEYWORDS

- Flat dysplasia • Dysplasia-associated lesions or masses
- Ulcerative colitis • Chromoendoscopy • Targeted biopsy

The increased risk for developing colorectal cancer (CRC) for patients with long-standing ulcerative colitis (UC) is well recognized.[1,2] To prevent the morbidity and mortality from CRC, it is essential to diagnose the lesions at the premalignant or early malignant stages. The findings of dysplasia[3] and dysplasia-associated lesions or masses (DALM)[4] are important in patients with UC because their findings often signify the presence of cancer.

Recent studies have shown that the detection of non-polypoid colorectal neoplasms (NP-CRN) is an integral component in the early detection of UC-associated CRC.[5] Unlike DALM, which is readily visible, NP-CRN is often subtle and can be difficult to detect. NP-CRN in UC often presents as redness or a granular patch of mucosa, which may not be readily distinguishable from the surrounding inflamed mucosa. Magnifying chromoendoscopy can be useful to enhance our ability to detect NP-CRN and enable targeted biopsies and increase the detection rate of dysplasia/cancer.[6,7] Within this perspective, the authors summarize the endoscopic diagnosis, prevalence, characteristics, and the recent concepts for management of NP-CRN in UC.

PREVALENCE OF NON-POLYPOID COLORECTAL NEOPLASMS IN ULCERATIVE COLITIS
Colorectal Cancer Risk in Patients with Ulcerative Colitis

The risk for developing CRC increases with early age at diagnosis of UC, longer duration of symptoms, and severity of inflammation and dysplasia.[8,9] In addition, postinflammatory polyps and strictures are features of previous severe inflammation and signify an increased risk for colorectal cancer.[10] A meta-analysis that reviewed 116

[a] Department of Endoscopy, Hiroshima University Hospital, 1-2-3 Kasumi, Minami-ku, Hiroshima 734-8551, Japan
[b] Department of Medicine and Molecular Science, Hiroshima University, 1-2-3 Kasumi, Minami-ku, Hiroshima 734-8551, Japan
* Corresponding author.
E-mail address: yueno@hiroshima-u.ac.jp

Gastrointest Endoscopy Clin N Am 20 (2010) 525–542
doi:10.1016/j.giec.2010.04.002
1052-5157/10/$ – see front matter © 2010 Elsevier Inc. All rights reserved.

studies of CRC in UC from around the world found the prevalence of CRC in subjects with UC to be 3.7% overall and 5.4% for those with pancolitis.[1] These incidence rates corresponded to cumulative probabilities of 2% by 10 years, 8% by 20 years, and 18% by 30 years. In a study sponsored by the Japanese Ministry of Health, Labor, and Welfare the prevalence is similar. The factors that increase the risk for developing CRC in the setting of UC are listed in **Box 1**.

PREVALENCE OF NON-POLYPOID COLORECTAL NEOPLASMS AMONG ULCERATIVE COLITIS-RELATED NEOPLASIAS

The prevalence of non-polypoid and polypoid lesions in UC varies to some degree. Sada and colleagues[11] reported that during the follow-up of 1115 subjects with UC, 39 lesions (31 subjects) of inflammatory bowel diseases (IBD)-related neoplasia were detected and 30% of dysplasias (6 of 20) were flat and 16% of colitic cancers (3 of 19) were depressed lesions. Toruner and colleagues[12] reported that among 635 subjects with IBD, 36 IBD-related dysplasias were found and 24 (66.7%) were flat and 12 (33.3%) were polypoid dysplasia. In a study of 110 neoplastic lesions in 56 subjects in a retrospective review of 525 subjects with IBD in the surveillance program, Rutter and colleagues[13] noted that 77% were macroscopically visible, with 23% flat. In the investigation by the Japanese Ministry of Health, Labor and, Welfare, 42 lesions (79%) were protruded, and 11 lesions (21%) were nonprotruded. In the authors' study of 1975 subjects with UC conducted at the Hiroshima University Hospital, 39 lesions of colorectal cancer/dysplasia were detected, 8 lesions (20.5%) of which were of the superficial type.

The variations in the epidemiology of NP-CRN in patients with UC might have arisen from the definition of flat dysplasia; some slightly elevated lesions might be classified as DALM instead of flat dysplasia. In addition, the rate of detection of NP-CRN in UC may also vary according to use of image enhancement and perhaps magnification. By using chromoscopy and magnification 4.75-fold more neoplasias could be detected than with conventional colonoscopy,[14] most are flat dysplasias. The presence of visible flat dysplastic lesions might be higher than expected. Hurlstone and colleagues[15] reported that magnification colonoscopy improves the detection of intraepithelial neoplasia in the endoscopic screening of patients with UC. They showed that 20 intraepithelial neoplastic lesions were detected from 12,850 nontargeted biopsies in the magnification group, whereas 49 intraepithelial neoplastic lesions were detected from the 644 targeted biopsies taken in the magnification group. This study showed

---

Box 1
Factors associated with increased risk of colorectal cancer in ulcerative colitis

Long duration of colitis

Extensive colonic involvement

Family history of colorectal cancer

Primary sclerosing cholangitis

Young age of inflammatory bowel diseases (IBD) onset

Backwash ileitis

Severity of inflammation

Strictures

that the prevalence of dysplasia indeed varies whether targeted or random biopsies were performed.

THE DETECTION AND DIAGNOSIS OF NON-POLYPOID COLORECTAL NEOPLASMS IN ULCERATIVE COLITIS
Bowel Preparations

Clean bowel preparation is critical. Without one, it is difficult to detect NP-CRN or to perform image-enhanced endoscopy when NP-CRN is detected.[16] In the authors' unit, they typically use 2 L polyethylene glycol solution or 1.8 L magnesium citrate immediately before the examination. These preparations do not induce inflammation. The authors ask that patients consume a low-residue diet the day before the procedure.

Detection of Non-Polypoid Colorectal Neoplasms in Ulcerative Colitis

Morphologically, NP-CRNs appear to be slightly elevated, completely flat, or slightly depressed as compared with the surrounding mucosa.[16] The term flat dysplasia is often used to describe slightly elevated lesions as the completely flat (0-IIb) or depressed (0-IIc) lesions are exceedingly rare.[17] The authors have summarized the suspicious findings that may represent the presence of NP-CRN in UC in **Box 2**.

The detection of NP-CRNs is performed with standard endoscopy by looking at the colonic mucosa for features of NP-CRN: slight color differentiation, friability, folds convergence, absence of vascular pattern, unevenness or mucosal deformity, or wall deformity.[18] Flat lesions may appear slightly reddish or pale,[5] although reddish finding is one of the most important clues in the detection of flat dysplasia.[11] The authors have included some examples of the appearance of NP-CRN in UC in **Figs. 1–4**. **Figs. 1** and **3** are examples of flat dysplasia in UC, which was detected according to redness. The redness of the dysplasia in UC often has a clear demarcation, which differentiates it from inflammation. In addition, flat elevations and nodular or granular mucosa are important factors in the recognition of dysplasia. As in **Fig. 2**, focal friability is also important for the detection of dysplasia. To identify these lesions, a colonoscopy should generally be performed at the quiescent stage because it is difficult to differentiate dysplastic lesions from inflammatory lesions.[19] As in **Fig. 4**, some lesions are well defined at the active stage.

IMAGE ENHANCED ENDOSCOPY
Dye-Based Image Enhanced Endoscopy

High-resolution colonoscopy with magnifying observation is useful for the detection and diagnosis of NP-CRN[20] and assessment of disease activity. In the authors' unit,

---

Box 2
Suspicious endoscopically visible alterations of NP-CRN in UC

Slightly elevated lesion

Focal friability

Obscure vascular pattern

Discoloration (uneven redness)

Villous mucosa (velvety appearance)

Irregular nodularity

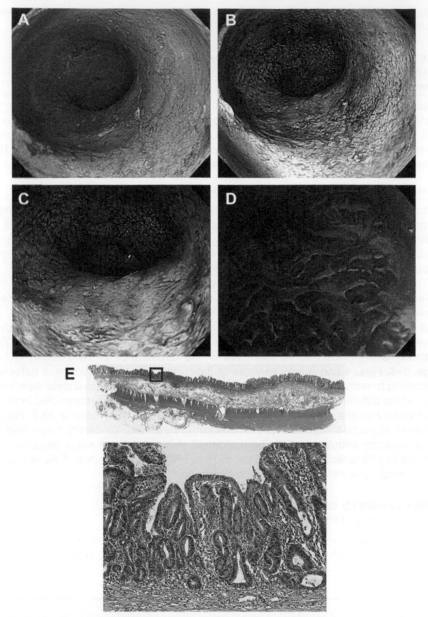

Fig. 1. (*A*) Conventional, non-chromoscopic view of the rectum. Note the lesions with red mucosal irregularity. (*B*) The same colonic segment following local application of a 0.5% indigo carmine solution (original magnification ×20). Note the focal lesion that is not covered with the indigo carmine solution. (*C*) The lesion is slightly elevated with mucous. (*D*) Crystal violet (0.05%) chromoscopy was applied to the lesion and high-magnification imaging acquired. The magnification imaging shows a Kudo type Vi crypt pattern. (*E*) Colectomy was performed and the lesion was histologically diagnosed as well-differentiated adenocarcinoma.

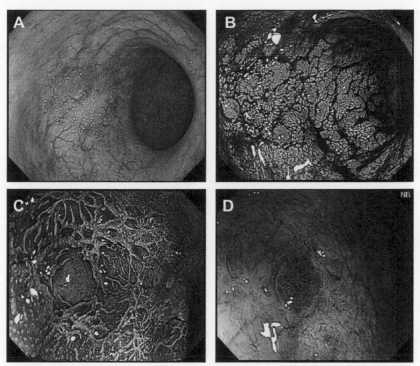

Fig. 2. (*A*) Conventional, non-chromoscopic view of the rectum. Note the subtle mucosal pallor with granular appearance. (*B*) The same colonic segment following local application of a 0.5% indigo carmine solution. Note the extensive flat mucosal change that was not visualized using conventional imaging. (*C*) Crystal violet (0.05%) chromoscopy was applied to the lesion and high-magnification imaging acquired at the central nodule. The magnification imaging shows a Kudo type Vi crypt pattern. (*D*) NBI shows a Hirata-Tanaka classification C3 pattern. This lesion was a well differentiated adenocarcinoma.

they typically perform high magnification colonoscopy with image enhancement only after they detect a suspicious lesion. They use the water jet to clean the area of interest from mucous or debris[21] and apply the dye for magnification endoscopy.

Other investigators, however, have used image enhancement to improve the detection of subtle colonic lesions.[7] Indigo carmine solution enhances the visualization of surface topography of the lesion and surrounding mucosa.[22] Kiesslich and colleagues reported 165 subjects with long-standing UC who were randomized to conventional colonoscopy or colonoscopy with chromoendoscopy using 0.1% methylene blue. More targeted biopsies were possible and significant intraepithelial neoplasia was detected in the chromoendoscopy group (32 vs 10; $P = .003$).[23] Rutter and colleagues[24] reported the importance of indigo carmine dye spraying for the detection of dysplasia in UC. They emphasized that no dysplasia was detected in 2904 nontargeted biopsies, but a targeted biopsy with pan-colonic chromoendoscopy required fewer biopsies and detected 9 dysplastic lesions, 7 of which were only visible after indigo carmine application. They concluded that the routine use of indigo carmine dye spray throughout the whole colon is simple, feasible, and safe. Hurlstone and colleagues[15] also emphasized that indigo carmine-assisted high magnification

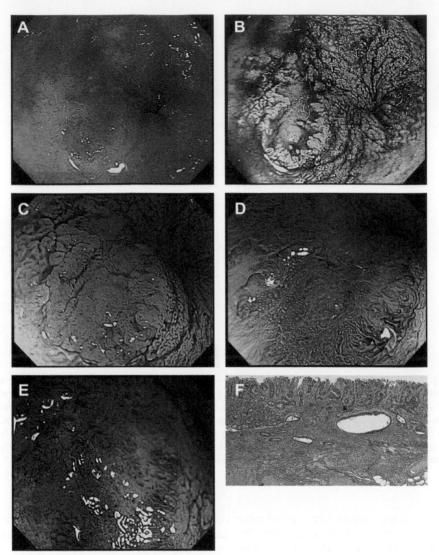

Fig. 3. (*A*) Conventional endoscopic view of the posterior rectum. Note the focal erythema. (*B*) The same lesion, now well demarcated after the local application of 0.5% indigo carmine solution (non-magnified view). (*C*) High-magnification imaging shows a Kudo type Vi pit pattern. (*D*) Crystal violet (0.05%) chromoscopy with high-magnification shows a Kudo type Vi crypt pattern. (*E*) NBI shows a Hirata-Tanaka classification C3 pattern. (*F*) Colectomy was performed and this lesion was an invasive adenocarcinoma.

chromoscopic colonoscopy improved the detection of intraepithelial neoplasia in the endoscopic screening of patients with UC.

Equipment-Based Image Enhanced Endoscopy

The authors have reported that narrow band imaging (NBI)[25] magnification is useful for the prediction of histologic diagnosis and invasion depth of colorectal tumors[26,27] in

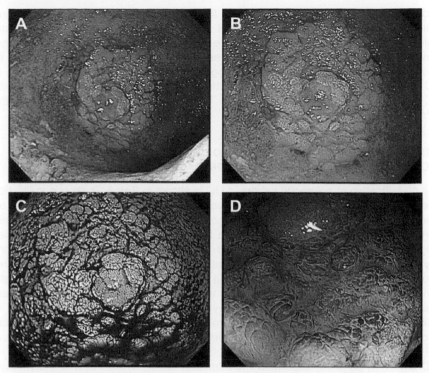

Fig. 4. (A, B) High-definition white light endoscopy of the rectum in a patient with long-standing UC. This mucosal area is highlighted as a pale granular lesion at the active stage of inflammation. (C) Indigo carmine 0.5% chromoscopy has been applied to the mucosa. A clearly defined flat, depressed lesion is delineated. (D) Crystal violet (0.05%) chromoscopy with high-magnification imaging shows a Kudo type Vi crypt pattern. Final diagnosis was of a high-grade dysplastic intraepithelial neoplastic lesion.

noncolitic colons. East and colleagues[28] extended the use of NBI in colitis surveillance and found that dysplastic lesions seen with NBI had a stronger (blacker) capillary vascular pattern compared with normal mucosa. Matsumoto and colleagues[29] reported that the tortuous pattern of capillaries determined by NBI colonoscopy might be a clue for the identification of dysplasia during surveillance for UC. Thus, NBI could be a useful additional method for distinguishing dysplastic from nondysplastic mucosa in UC.

Autofluorescence imaging (AFI) in endoscopy has been reported to be promising for the detection of dysplasia in UC,[30,31] although the clinical potential of AFI in routine endoscopic practice has been complicated by high false-positive detection rates, particularly in cases of flat mucosal disease.

PIT PATTERNS IN NON-POLYPOID COLORECTAL NEOPLASMS IN ULCERATIVE COLITIS

After dye spraying, the authors evaluate the pit pattern of the mucosal surface.[32] The current pit-pattern classification, however, may not be completely applicable in UC. The main pit patterns of dysplasia or early colitic cancer were type IV and type IIIS with IIIL.[15] Sada and colleagues[11] described that 10 protruded lesions of dysplasia and 5 early cancers showed IIIS- to IIIL-type pits or IV-type pits. Hata and colleagues[33] showed that the type I pit pattern corresponded to nondysplastic lesions, whereas type III, IV, and V pit patterns correspond well to dysplastic lesions. However, they also noted that some nonneoplastic flat lesions also have III and IV pits. This is because the pit pattern of regenerative hyperplastic villous mucosa in UC is difficult to distinguish from neoplastic pit patterns as the pits in patients with UC can become elongated or irregular depending on the improvement in the inflammation.[20]

DIFFERENTIATION OF NON-POLYPOID COLORECTAL NEOPLASMS FROM DYSPLASIA-ASSOCIATED LESIONS OR MASSES

The classification of colorectal tumors in UC is shown in **Box 3**. Dysplasia in UC has been classified macroscopically as elevated or flat, depending respectively on whether or not it corresponds to an endoscopically visible lesion.[34] Elevated lesions, conventionally referred to by the acronym DALM span a broad gamut that includes single and multiple polyps, bumps, plaques, and velvety patches (**Fig. 5**).[4,35] Traditionally, flat dysplasia is detected microscopically in random biopsy specimens from unremarkable mucosa. Because most dysplasia have been thought to be macroscopically invisible, multiple nontargeted biopsies were recommended for cancer surveillance.[34,36] However, recent papers revealed that most dysplasia in UC is visible.[13,37,38] This is because of improvements in endoscopic resolution rather than a change in the biology of these tumors. The differences between DALM and NP-CRN are listed in **Box 4**.

DALMs may be further separated into adenoma-like (ALD) lesions, which have a low risk for progression to carcinoma, and nonadenoma-like (NALD) lesions, which have a high rate of neoplastic progression.[39] ALD has been defined at endomicroscopy as any lesional morphology within or outside of a colitis zone with no adjacent flat neoplastic architecture.[40] NALD has been defined as any lesional morphology within a colitis zone accompanied by adjacent mucosal neoplastic criteria (**Fig. 6**). The differential diagnosis of ALD and NALD is important because NALD is considered to be an indication for colectomy, whereas ALD is considered appropriate for polypectomy.[41–43]

Box 3
Endoscopic appearances of flat and elevated lesions in UC

NP-CRN

  Slightly elevated

  Completely flat

  Slightly depressed

Polypoid CRN

  Nonadenoma-like DALM

  Adenoma-like DALM

Inflammatory lesions

  Nonneoplastic flat lesions

  Inflammatory polyps

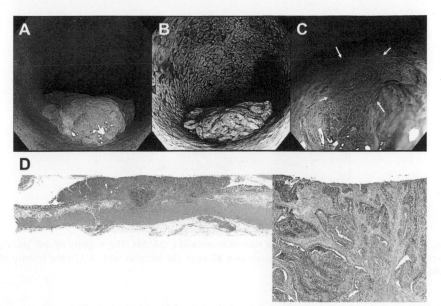

Fig. 5. Colonoscopic and histological findings in a case of DALM. (*A*) Conventional colonoscopy shows a flat-topped elevation in the sigmoid colon. (*B*) The same colonic segment following local application of a 0.5% indigo carmine solution. (*C*) Crystal violet (0.05%) chromoscopy was applied to the lesion and high-magnification imaging acquired at the central slight depression. A VN crypt pattern is evident. (*D*) Histology revealed that the lesion was a moderately differentiated adenocarcinoma associated with an adenoma, pSM2, ly0, v0, HM0, VM0.

DIFFERENTIATION OF NON-POLYPOID COLORECTAL NEOPLASMS FROM FLAT NONNEOPLASTIC LESIONS

It is recommended that identification of flat dysplasia in UC should be performed at the quiescent stage and such lesions should be sampled for biopsies. This recommendation is because the differentiation of flat dysplastic lesion can be difficult to differentiate from inflammatory mucosa[44] even when the disease is quiescent as the pit pattern of the nonneoplastic mucosa can include various types, such as I, II, IIIL, or

Box 4		
Differentiation of DALM and NP-CRN		
Tumors	**DALM**	**NP-CRN**
Prevalence (%)	60–70	30–40
Low-grade dysplasia/high-grade dysplasia	LGD<HGD	LGD>HGD
Endoscopy	Visible	Difficult to see
Pit pattern	IIIL–V	IIIL–Vi
NBI	Tortuous	Honeycomb/villous/tortuous
Differential diagnosis	Inflammatory polyps adenoma-like DALM	Inflammatory flat lesions

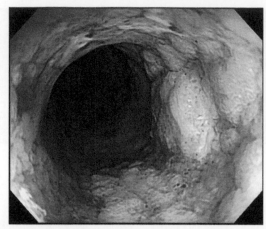

Fig. 6. Endoscopic images showing a non-adenoma-like DALMs. The slightly raised, poorly circumscribed dysplastic lesion was seen in a 38-year-old woman with a 17-year history of total colitis.

IV. Kiesslich and colleagues[23] reported that 6 of the detected 86 nonneoplastic mucosal lesions showed the III-V pit pattern. Matsumoto and colleagues[29] reported that in 46 subjects with UC, 276 areas of flat mucosa were surveyed and only 3 of these lesions were diagnosed as dysplasia.

The authors have found that about a half of the flat lesions in UC are nonneoplastic inflammatory lesions (**Fig. 7**). Immunohistochemistry with p53 may help to differentiate these lesions.[45] In the future, molecular and biomarkers may improve the identification of dysplastic changes by assessing telomere length, anaphase bridges, and chromosomal in situ hybridization.[46]

MANAGEMENT OF NON-POLYPOID COLORECTAL NEOPLASMS IN ULCERATIVE COLITIS
Histologic Classification of Dysplasia in Ulcerative Colitis

The management of NP-CRN in UC is an area with differing opinions.[47,48] It depends on whether NP-CRN is unifocal or multifocal, or whether the histology reveals low- or high-grade dysplasia. The histologic classification of dysplasia in IBD is based on a 1983 consensus report in which a group of expert gastrointestinal pathologists proposed classifying biopsy specimens into 5 categories: negative for dysplasia; indefinite for dysplasia; and positive for low-grade dysplasia (LGD), high-grade dysplasia (HGD), or invasive cancer.[49] Dysplasia is defined as an unequivocal neoplastic proliferation of the epithelium that is confined to the mucosal layer and graded as high or low. The distinction between low- and high-grade dysplasia depends on the distribution of nuclei within the cells; low-grade dysplasia is characterized by nuclei that remain confined to the basal half of the cells and high-grade dysplasia by nuclei that are stratified haphazardly between the basal and apical halves.[49]

Unifocal flat low-grade dysplasia
Several studies reported a 50% rate of progression from LGD to more advanced neoplasia (either HGD or CRC) over 5 years.[3,50–54] Ullman and colleagues[53] remarked that the presence of flat LGD was a powerful predictor of advanced neoplasia and that continued surveillance as opposed to immediate colectomy was "at best a risky

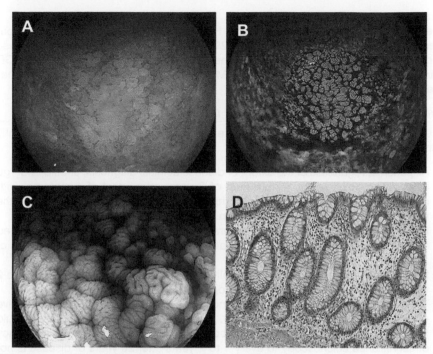

Fig. 7. Superficial flat lesions in the setting of UC. (*A*) Initial view of the lesion. Close-up (*B*) indigo carmine spray. (*C*) Magnification imaging (×100) shows a Kudo type IIIL crypt pattern. (*D*) No dysplasia was found histologically.

strategy." Data from St Mark's Hospital indicate that the 5-year cumulative probability of progressing from LGD to HGD or cancer is 54%. Coexisting CRC was found in 20% of subjects with LGD undergoing colectomy, and 39.1% of subjects with LGD progressed to HGD or CRC during follow-up.[3]

There are, however, critics to the previously mentioned reports, who believe that their recommendations lead to over treatment in many patients. Lim and colleagues[55] demonstrated that only 3 of 29 (10%) subjects with LGD progressed to HGD or cancer after 10 years. They concluded that LGD is insufficient to justify colectomy. Befrits and colleagues[56] reported on a series of 60 subjects with LGD, in whom there was no progression to CRC, and observed only 2 cases of HGD in dysplasia-associated lesions or masses over a mean follow-up of 10 years. These variations might come from the difficulty in the diagnosis of LGD because of histologically active inflammation. Based on these reports, if flat LGD is identified, either colectomy or repeat surveillance should be considered. If colectomy is not performed, then obviously close endoscopic and clinical follow-up should be performed to determine that the lesion has been completely removed and no metachronous lesions arise.

Multifocal flat low-grade dysplasia
If multifocal flat LGDs are found, a colectomy should be seriously considered.[48,57] The Crohn's and Colitis Foundation of America (CCFA) consensus strongly recommends a proctocolectomy if multifocal flat LGD, repetitive flat LGD, or more advanced dysplasia is found during subsequent surveillance colonoscopies.[58] If patients decide against a proctocolectomy, repeat surveillance examinations should be undertaken within 3 to 6 months or less.

Flat high-grade dysplasia

There is little controversy surrounding flat HGD because colectomy specimens from these patients have concurrent CRC in 42% to 45.5% of cases.[3,59] Based on these and related studies, strong agreement therefore exists that the presence of HGD warrants prompt proctocolectomy.[3,58–60] Management of dysplasia in UC is summarized in **Fig. 8**.

Guidelines in Surveillance Colonoscopy in Ulcerative Colitis

The guidelines of the American Gastroenterological Association[61] that were recently published include

1. All patients, regardless of the extent of disease at initial diagnosis, should undergo a screening colonoscopy a maximum of 8 years after onset of symptoms, with multiple biopsy specimens obtained throughout the entire colon, to assess the true microscopic extent of inflammation.
2. Patients with ulcerative proctitis or ulcerative proctosigmoiditis are not considered at increased risk for IBD-related CRC and thus may be managed on the basis of average-risk recommendations.
3. Patients with extensive or left-sided colitis should begin surveillance within 1 to 2 years after the initial screening endoscopy.
4. The optimal surveillance interval has not been clearly defined. After 2 negative examinations (no dysplasia or cancer), further surveillance examinations should be performed every 1 to 3 years. Recent data suggest that increasing the frequency of surveillance colonoscopy to every 1 to 2 years after 20 years of disease is not needed for all patients, but should be individualized according to the presence or absence of other risk factors.
5. There are no prospective studies that have determined the optimal number of biopsy specimens that should be obtained to detect dysplasia reliably.

Management of dysplasia in UC

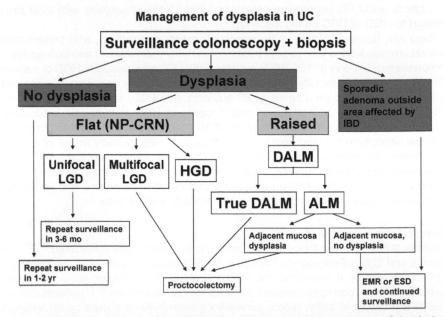

Fig. 8. Algorithm for screening/surveillance for CRC in UC and management of dysplasia.

Representative biopsy specimens from each anatomic section of the colon are recommended. One study has recommended that a minimum of 33 biopsy specimens be taken in patients with pancolitis.
6. Patients with primary sclerosing cholangitis (PSC) should begin surveillance colonoscopy at the time of this diagnosis and then undergo yearly colonoscopy thereafter.
7. Ideally, surveillance colonoscopy should be performed when the colonic disease is in remission.
8. Patients with a history of CRC in first-degree relatives; ongoing active endoscopic or histologic inflammation; or anatomic abnormalities, such as a foreshortened colon, stricture, or multiple inflammatory pseudopolyps may benefit from more frequent surveillance examinations.
9. These recommendations also apply to patients with Crohn's colitis who have disease involving at least one-third of the length of the colon.

The British Society for Gastroenterology recommendations,[62] although published earlier, are more progressive and perhaps reflect the literature more closely in regards to the utility of use of image enhancement to direct biopsy rather than random biopsy (see no. 4 discussed later). Their guidelines include

1. All patients with UC or Crohn's colitis should undergo a screening colonoscopy approximately 10 years after the onset of colitic symptoms to assess disease extent and other endoscopic risk factors.
2. Surveillance colonoscopies should be performed, where possible, when the disease is in remission. However, a surveillance procedure should not be unduly delayed if remission cannot be achieved.
3. The risk for cancer is influenced by the duration and extent of disease and additional risk factors (eg, PSC and family history of CRC), and is also linked to the endoscopic and histologic appearances at colonoscopy. The screening intervals recommended account for such variables. Surveillance colonoscopies should be conducted yearly, every 3 years, or every 5 years, accordingly.
4. Pan-colonic dye spraying with targeted biopsy of abnormal areas is recommended. If chromoendoscopy is not used, 2 to 4 random biopsy specimens from every 10 cm of colon should be taken, with additional biopsy specimens of suspicious areas.
5. It is not necessary to recommend colectomy if a polyp is detected within an area of inflammation and can be removed in its entirety.

The British Society guidelines also recognized that flat dysplastic lesions and adenoma-like masses in UC could be managed safely by endoscopic mucosal resection (EMR).[63,64] Hurlstone and colleagues[63] reported that a total of 82 flat lesions underwent EMR, 2 of which could not be resected endoscopically because of nonlifting at submucosal injection. Recently, colorectal endoscopic submucosal dissection (ESD) has been increasingly used as a therapeutic method for early colorectal tumors, especially for laterally spreading tumors.[65,66] ESD may also be indicated for non-polypoid lesions in UC because the lesions may be accompanied by submucosal fibrosis, which would result in insufficient submucosal elevation with hyaluronate sodium. ESD is also useful for the diagnosis of colorectal tumors in UC, especially flat lesions, because it is sometimes difficult to distinguish them from benign lesions. **Fig. 9** shows a flat lesion in a 65-year-old woman. The lesion with submucosal fibrosis was successfully resected by ESD. Post-ESD resection histopathology showed a serrated adenoma. ESD, instead of multiple biopsies in UC, may be useful not

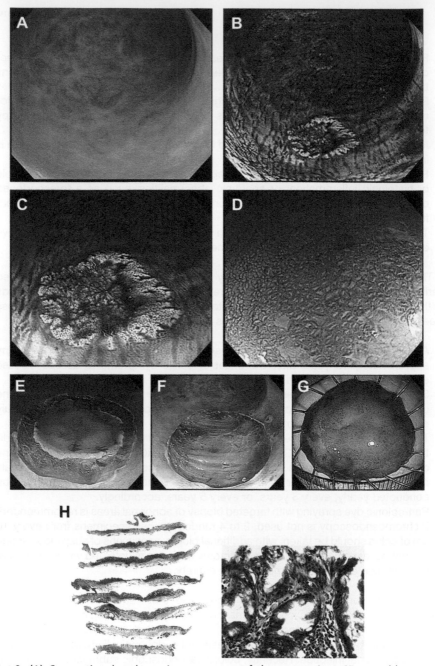

Fig. 9. (A) Conventional endoscopic appearance of the rectum in a 65-year-old woman. Note the focal round-shaped lesion at the bottom on the inactive mucosa with multiple ulcer scars. (B) Mucosal appearance after chromoscopy with indigo carmine 0.5%. A IIa+IIc lesion is now clearly delineated. (C) High-magnification chromoscopic images of the lesion at magnification ×100. (D) Crystal violet (0.05%) chromoscopy was applied to the lesion and high-magnification imaging acquired at the central slight depression. A II pit pattern is evident. (E) The lesion was treated by ESD. A circumferential incision was undertaken. (F) The mucosal defect after post endoscopic dissection, with successful vertical plane dissection to the muscularis layer. See the associated blue stranding of the muscularis layer with indigo carmine chromoscopy. (G) Resected mucosa resected by ESD. (H) Histology revealed that the lesion was a serrated adenoma.

only for the treatment of sporadic localized adenomatous lesions but also for the diagnosis of dysplasia, and would also minimize the sampling error.

SUMMARY

The incidence of colorectal cancer associated with UC increases with time. It is imperative to identify DALM and NP-CRN to reduce the morbidity and mortality from colorectal cancer associated with UC. In the past, NP-CRN in UC has only been considered as detectable in random biopsy specimens from unremarkable mucosa examined microscopically. Recent findings, however, suggest most dysplastic lesions in UC can be considered visible under careful endoscopic observation. To find NP-CRN in UC, careful examination of well-prepared mucosa and noting subtle differences is necessary. Magnifying chromoendoscopy, therefore, can be useful to endoscopically diagnose these subtle findings. The authors believe that targeted biopsies during chromoendoscopy will increasingly be used and replace random biopsies in the future. EMR and ESD may be included in the management paradigm for surveillance of NP-CRN in UC, although prospective studies fully addressing this point are needed.

REFERENCES

1. Eaden JA, Abrams KR, Mayberry JF, et al. The risk of colorectal cancer in ulcerative colitis: a meta-analysis. Gut 2001;48:526–35.
2. Bernstein CN. Ulcerative colitis with low-grade dysplasia. Gastroenterology 2004; 127:950–6.
3. Rutter MD, Saunders BP, Wilkinson KH, et al. Thirty year after analysis of a colonoscopic surveillance program for neoplasia in ulcerative colitis. Gastroenterology 2006;130:1030–8.
4. Blackstone MU, Riddle RF, Rogers BH, et al. Dysplasia-associated lesion or mass (DALM) detected by colonoscopy in long-standing ulcerative colitis; an indication for colectomy. Gastroenterology 1981;80:366–74.
5. Nagasako K, Iizuka B, Ishii F, et al. Colonoscopic diagnosis of dysplasia and early cancer in longstanding colitis. J Gastroenterol 1995;30(Suppl VIII):36–9.
6. Kiesslich R, Neurath M. Chromo- and magnifying endoscopy for colorectal lesions. Eur J Gastroenterol Hepatol 2005;17:793–801.
7. Hurlstone DP. The detection of flat and depressed colorectal lesions: which endoscopic imaging approach? Gastroenterology 2008;135:338–43.
8. Rutter MD, Saunders BP, Wilkinson KH, et al. Severity of inflammation is a risk factor for progression to colorectal neoplasia in ulcerative colitis. Gastroenterology 2004;126:451–9.
9. Gupta RB, Harpaz N, Itzkowitz S, et al. Histologic inflammation is a risk factor for progression to colorectal neoplasia in ulcerative colitis: a cohort study. Gastroenterology 2007;133:1099–105.
10. Rutter M, Saunders B, Wilkinson KH, et al. Cancer surveillance in longstanding ulcerative colitis: endoscopic appearances help predict cancer risk. Gut 2004; 53:1813–6.
11. Sada M, Igarashi M, Yoshizawa S, et al. Dye spraying and magnifying endoscopy for dysplasia and cancer surveillance in ulcerative colitis. Dis Colon Rectum 2004;47:1816–23.
12. Toruner M, Harewood GC, Loftus EV Jr, et al. Endoscopic factors in the diagnosis of colorectal dysplasia in chronic inflammatory bowel disease. Inflamm Bowel Dis 2005;11:428–34.

13. Rutter MD, Saunders BP, Wilkinson KH, et al. Most dysplasia in ulcerative colitis is visible at colonoscopy. Gastrointest Endosc 2004;60:334–9.
14. Kiesslich R, Goetz M, Lammersdorf K, et al. Chromoscopy-guided endomicroscopy increases the diagnostic yield of intraepithelial neoplasia in ulcerative colitis. Gastroenterology 2007;132:874–82.
15. Hurlstone DP, Sanders DS, Lobo AJ, et al. Indigo carmine-assisted high-magnification chromoscopic colonoscopy for the detection and characterization of intraepithelial neoplasia in ulcerative colitis: a prospective evaluation. Endoscopy 2005;37:1186–92.
16. Soetikno R, Friedland S, Kaltenbach T, et al. Nonpolypoid (flat and depressed) colorectal neoplasms. Gastroenterology 2006;130:566–76.
17. Kudo S, Lambert R, Allen JI, et al. Nonpolypoid neoplastic lesions of the colorectal mucosa. Gastrointest Endosc 2008;68:S3–47.
18. Tanaka S, Kaltenbach T, Chayama K, et al. High-magnification colonoscopy. Gastrointest Endosc 2006;64:604–13.
19. Matsumoto T, Iwao Y, Igarashi M, et al. Endoscopic and chromoendoscopic atlas featuring dysplastic lesions in surveillance colonoscopy for patients with long-standing ulcerative colitis. Inflamm Bowel Dis 2008;14:259–64.
20. Kunihiro M, Tanaka S, Sumii M, et al. Magnifying endoscopic features of ulcerative colitis reflect histologic inflammation. Inflamm Bowel Dis 2004;10:737–44.
21. Seitz U, Seewald S, Bohnacker S, et al. Advances in interventional gastrointestinal endoscopy in colon and rectum. Int J Colorectal Dis 2003;18:12–8.
22. Fujii T, Hasegawa RT, Saitoh Y, et al. Chromoscopy during colonoscopy. Endoscopy 2001;33:1036–41.
23. Kiesslich R, Fritch J, Holtmann M, et al. Methylene-blue aided chromoendoscopy for the detection of intraepithelial neoplasia and colon cancer in ulcerative colitis. Gastroenterology 2003;124:880–8.
24. Rutter MD, Saunders BP, Schofield G, et al. Pancolonic indigo carmine dye spraying for the detection of dysplasia in ulcerative colitis. Gut 2004;53:256–60.
25. Gono K, Obi T, Yamaguchi M, et al. Appearance of enhanced tissue features on narrow-band endoscopic imaging. J Biomed Opt 2004;9:568–77.
26. Hirata M, Tanaka S, Oka S, et al. Evaluations of microvessels in colorectal tumors by narrow band imaging magnification. Gastrointest Endosc 2007;66:945–52.
27. Kanao H, Tanaka S, Oka S, et al. Narrow-band imaging magnification predicts the histology and invasion depth of colorectal tumors. Gastrointest Endosc 2009;69:631–6.
28. East JE, Suzuki N, von Herbay A, et al. Narrow band imaging with magnification for dysplasia detection and pit pattern assessment in ulcerative colitis surveillance: a case with multiple dysplasia associated lesions or masses. Gut 2006;55:1432–5.
29. Matsumoto T, Kudo T, Jo Y, et al. Magnifying colonoscopy with narrow band imaging system for the diagnosis of dysplasia in ulcerative colitis: a pilot study. Gastrointest Endosc 2007;66:957–65.
30. Ochsenkuhn T, Tillack C, Stepp H, et al. Low frequency of colorectal dysplasia in patients with long-standing inflammatory bowel disease colitis: detection by fluorescence endoscopy. Endoscopy 2006;38:477–82.
31. Matsumoto T, Moriyama T, Yao T, et al. Autofluorescence imaging colonoscopy for the diagnosis of dysplasia in ulcerative colitis. Inflamm Bowel Dis 2007;13:640–1.

32. Kudo S, Rubio CA, Teixeira CR, et al. Pit pattern in colorectal neoplasia: endoscopic magnifying view. Endoscopy 2001;33:367–73.
33. Hata K, Watanabe T, Motoi T, et al. Pitfalls of pit pattern diagnosis in ulcerative colitis-associated dysplasia. Gastroenterology 2004;126:374–6.
34. Tytgat GNJ, Dhir V, Gopinath N. Endoscopic appearance of dysplasia and cancer in inflammatory bowel disease. Eur J Cancer 1995;31:1174–7.
35. Butt JH, Konishi F, Morson BC, et al. Macroscopic lesions in dysplasia and carcinoma complicating ulcerative colitis. Dig Dis Sci 1983;28:18–26.
36. Sharan R, Scoen RE. Cancer in inflammatory bowel disease. An evidence-based analysis and guide for physicians and patients. Gastroenterol Clin North Am 2002;31:237–54.
37. Rubin DT, Rothe JA, Hetzel JT, et al. Are dysplasia and colorectal cancer endoscopically visible in patients with ulcerative colitis? Gastrointest Endosc 2007;65: 998–1004.
38. Blonski W, Kundu R, Lewis J, et al. Is dysplasia visible during surveillance colonoscopy in patients with ulcerative colitis? Scand J Gastroenterol 2008;43: 698–703.
39. Odze RD. Adenomas and adenoma-like DALMs in chronic ulcerative colitis: a clinical, pathological, and molecular review. Am J Gastroenterol 1999;94: 1746–50.
40. Suzuki K, Muto T, Shinozaki M, et al. Differential diagnosis of dysplasia-associated lesion or mass and coincidental adenoma in ulcerative colitis. Dis Colon Rectum 1998;41:322–7.
41. Engelsgjerd M, Farraye FA, Odze RD. Polypectomy may be adequate treatment for adenoma-like dysplastic lesions in chronic ulcerative colitis. Gastroenterology 1999;117:1288–94.
42. Odze RD, Farraye FA, Hecht JL, et al. Long-term follow-up after polypectomy treatment for adenoma-like dysplastic lesions in ulcerative colitis. Clin Gastroenterol Hepatol 2004;2:534–41.
43. Vieth M, Behrens H, Stolte M. Sporadic adenoma in ulcerative colitis: endoscopic resection is an adequate treatment. Gut 2006;55:1151–5.
44. Fujiya M, Saitoh Y, Nomura M, et al. Minute findings by magnifying colonoscopy are useful for the evaluation of ulcerative colitis. Gastrointest Endosc 2002;56: 535–42.
45. Wong NACS, Harrison DJ. Colorectal neoplasia in ulcerative colitis-recent advances. Histopathology 2001;39:221–34.
46. Bronner MP, O'Sullivan JN, Pabinovitch PS, et al. Genomic biomarkers to improve ulcerative colitis neoplasia surveillance. Am J Pathol 2008;173:1853–69.
47. Mitchell PJ, Salmo E, Haboubi NY. Inflammatory bowel disease: the problems of dysplasia and surveillance. Tech Coloproctol 2007;11:299–309.
48. Itzkowitz SH, Harpaz N. Diagnosis and management of dysplasia in patients with inflammatory bowel diseases. Gastroenterology 2004;126:1634–48.
49. Riddell RH, Goldman H, Ransohoff DF, et al. Dysplasia in inflammatory bowel disease: standardized classification with provisional clinical applications. Hum Pathol 1983;14:931–68.
50. Connell WR, Lennard-Jones JE, Williams CB, et al. Factors affecting the outcome of endoscopic surveillance for cancer in ulcerative colitis. Gastroenterology 1994; 107:934–44.
51. Linberg B, Perrson B, Veress B, et al. Twenty years' colonoscopic surveillance of patients with ulcerative colitis. Detection of dysplastic and malignant transformation. Scand J Gastroenterol 1996;31:1195–204.

52. Ullman TA, Loftus EV Jr, Kakar S, et al. The fate of low grade dysplasia in ulcerative colitis. Am J Gastroenterol 2002;97:922–7.
53. Ullman T, Croog V, Harpaz N, et al. Progression of flat low-grade dysplasia to advanced neoplasia in patients with ulcerative colitis. Gastroenterology 2003; 125:1311–9.
54. Goldblum JR. The histologic diagnosis of dysplasia, dysplasia-associated lesion or mass, and adenoma: a pathologist's perspective. J Clin Gastroenterol 2003;36: S63–9.
55. Lim DH, Dixon MF, Vail A, et al. Ten year follow up of ulcerative colitis patients with and without low-grade dysplasia. Gut 2003;52:1127–32.
56. Befrits R, Ljung T, Jaramillo E, et al. Low-grade dysplasia in extensive, long-standing inflammatory bowel disease. Dis Colon Rectum 2002;45:615–20.
57. Ahmadi A, Polyak S, Draganov PV. Colorectal cancer surveillance in inflammatory bowel disease: the search continues. World J Gastroenterol 2009;15:61–6.
58. Itzkowitz SH, Present DH. Consensus conference: colorectal cancer screening and surveillance in inflammatory bowel disease. Inflamm Bowel Dis 2005;11: 314–21.
59. Bernstein CN, Shanahan F, Weinstein WM, et al. Are we telling patients the truth about surveillance colonoscopy in ulcerative colitis? Lancet 1994;343:71–4.
60. Rodriguez SA, Collins JM, Knigge KL, et al. Surveillance and management of dysplasia in ulcerative colitis. Gastrointest Endosc 2007;65:432–9.
61. Farraye FA, Odze RD, Eaden J, et al. AGA technical review on the diagnosis and management of colorectal neoplasia in inflammatory bowel disease. Gastroenterology 2010;138:746–74.
62. Eaden J, Mayberry JF, British Society for Gastroenterology, et al. Guidelines for screening and surveillance of asymptomatic colorectal cancer in patients with inflammatory bowel disease. Gut 2002;51(Suppl V):v10–2.
63. Hurlstone DP, Sanders DS, Atkinson R, et al. Endoscopic mucosal resection for flat neoplasia in chronic ulcerative colitis: can we change the endoscopic management paradigm? Gut 2007;56:838–46.
64. Smith L-A, Baraza W, Tiffin N, et al. Endoscopic resection of adenoma-like mass in chronic ulcerative colitis using a combined endoscopic mucosal resection and cap assisted submucosal dissection technique. Inflamm Bowel Dis 2008;14: 1380–6.
65. Tanaka S, Oka S, Chayama K, et al. Colorectal endoscopic submucosal dissection: present status and future prospective, including its differentiation from endoscopic mucosal resection. J Gastroenterol 2008;43:641–51.
66. Oka S, Tanaka S, Kanao H, et al. Therapeutic strategy for colorectal laterally spreading tumor. Dig Endosc 2009;21(Suppl 1):S43–6.

Serrated Adenoma: A Distinct Form of Non-Polypoid Colorectal Neoplasia?

Amy E. Noffsinger, MD[a],*, John Hart, MD[b]

KEYWORDS

• Hyperplastic polyp • Adenoma • Colorectal cancer
• Microsatellite instability • CpG island methylator phenotype

Until 20 years ago, 2 major forms of colorectal epithelial polyp were recognized: the adenoma and the hyperplastic polyp. Adenomas have long been accepted as neoplastic, precursor lesions for colorectal adenocarcinoma. In contrast, hyperplastic polyps were for the most part regarded as innocuous lesions without neoplastic potential. It was known that hyperplastic polyps could be identified adjacent to a significant percentage of colorectal adenomas,[1] and that they occur with higher frequency in populations at greater risk of developing colorectal cancer,[2] but they were nevertheless felt by most to represent nonneoplastic bystander lesions.

In 1990, however, this view of colorectal polyps was challenged when Longacre and Fenoglio-Preiser published a study[3] examining a group of polyps that showed mixed histologic features of hyperplastic and adenomatous polyps. These lesions were believed to represent not mixed tumors with 2 separate hyperplastic and adenomatous components, but a single entity in which the glands had a serrated architecture, and the cells lining them showed nuclear features reminiscent of adenoma. These lesions were termed serrated adenomas, but were felt by the investigators to represent a variant of villous or tubulovillous adenoma rather than a lesion related to hyperplastic polyps.

Subsequent scattered reports and small series of colorectal adenocarcinomas associated with giant or large hyperplastic polyps (usually defined as >1 cm), however, suggested that at least some hyperplastic polyps had malignant potential.[4,5]

[a] Department of Pathology, University of Cincinnati, PO Box 670529, 231 Albert Sabin Way, Cincinnati, OH 45267-0529, USA
[b] Department of Pathology, University of Chicago Medical Center, 5841 South Maryland Avenue MC6101, Chicago, IL 60637, USA
* Corresponding author.
E-mail address: amy.noffsinger@uc.edu

Gastrointest Endoscopy Clin N Am 20 (2010) 543–563
doi:10.1016/j.giec.2010.03.012
1052-5157/10/$ – see front matter © 2010 Elsevier Inc. All rights reserved.

giendo.theclinics.com

Adenocarcinomas were also reported arising in mixed hyperplastic and adenomatous polyps.[6] In addition, the presence of multiple hyperplastic polyps in the form of hyperplastic polyposis[7–9] was clearly associated with the development of colorectal adenocarcinoma.

The concept that the lesions previously categorized as hyperplastic polyps actually represented several distinct entities emerged with the work of Torlakovic and Snover.[9] These investigators showed that the polyps arising in patients with hyperplastic polyposis had morphologic features that were different from those of small sporadic hyperplastic polyps, and that these features could reliably be used to differentiate between the potentially precancerous polyps and those that probably did not pose a risk for progression to colorectal cancer. In 2003, this group studied a set of sporadic serrated lesions, and showed that several discrete types of sporadic serrated polyps were also identifiable, and that these polyps could generally be divided into those with abnormal proliferation, termed sessile serrated adenomas, and those with normal proliferation, termed hyperplastic polyps.[10]

MORPHOLOGIC FEATURES AND CLASSIFICATION OF SERRATED COLON POLYPS

As a result of the studies described earlier, it has become clear that not all serrated polyps merely represent innocuous hyperplastic polyps, but that these lesions comprise a heterogeneous group of polyps, some of which are likely associated with a significant cancer risk. The current classification of serrated colorectal polyps is summarized in **Box 1**.

ENDOSCOPIC FEATURES OF SERRATED POLYPS

Endoscopically, hyperplastic polyps typically appear pale and sessile, and may flatten with air insufflation. They are characteristically small (<5 mm) and are located in the distal colon.[11] Serrated adenomas may be of 2 macroscopic types: polypoid and nonpolypoid or superficial. Polypoid serrated adenomas tend to occur in the distal colon, and are usually smaller than their superficial counterparts.[12] Superficial serrated adenomas occur throughout the colon, but those arising on the right are often larger than those occurring elsewhere in the colon.[13] Small polypoid serrated adenomas usually appear as small pale nodules that are often intermingled with hyperplastic polyps, lesions that endoscopically have a similar appearance.[13] Larger polypoid

---

Box 1
Classification of serrated lesions of the colorectum

Hyperplastic polyps

   Goblet-cell rich variant

   Microvesicular variant

   Mucin-poor variant

Sessile serrated adenoma

Traditional serrated adenoma

Mixed polyps

Hyperplastic polyposis

Serrated carcinoma

serrated polyps are often lobulated and red, an appearance similar to that of traditional adenomatous polyps. Small flat serrated adenomas frequently appear as small whitish spots with ill-defined margins that are better visualized after being sprayed with dye. Large, flat serrated adenomas appear as white areas with a smooth, granular or nodular surface.[13] Some lesions show abundant surface mucus, and appear as bile-stained areas or thickened folds.

HISTOLOGIC FEATURES OF SERRATED POLYPS
Hyperplastic Polyps

True hyperplastic polyps comprise 80% to 90% of all serrated lesions, and likely have no neoplastic risk.[3,10,14] Histologically, the colonic glands comprising hyperplastic polyps appear serrated, but the serrated change is limited to the upper half of the crypt (**Fig. 1**). The degree of serration present is variable among individual lesions. The deeper crypts often show expansion of the proliferative zone, but are not dilated. They appear straight and tubular, similar to those observed in normal colonic crypts. The collagen table underlying the surface epithelium of hyperplastic polyps is often thickened.

Conventional hyperplastic polyps show an expanded, but symmetric proliferation zone as illustrated by Ki-67 (MIB-1) immunostaining.[15] In addition, cytokeratin 20 staining is retained in the upper portion of the colonic crypt in a pattern similar to that seen in normal colonic mucosa.[15]

Hyperplastic polyps may be subclassified into 3 types: microvesicular, goblet-cell rich and mucin-poor based on the mucin content of the epithelial cells.[10] Such subclassification has no clinical usefulness, but has interesting molecular biologic correlates (see later discussion). The microvesicular variant is the most common, and represents the typical hyperplastic polyp found in the distal colon. It is character-ized by vesicular mucin-containing epithelial cells, and numerous goblet cell abnor-malities. Overall, goblet cells are decreased in number compared with normal

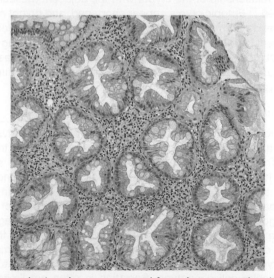

Fig. 1. This true hyperplastic polyp was removed from the rectum. The glands comprising it show prominent superficial serration. The nuclei are small and basally oriented. The cyto-plasm contains vesicular appearing mucin droplets.

colonic mucosa. Goblet-cell rich hyperplastic polyps commonly show less serration of the crypts than other hyperplastic polyp variants. Serration in this group of polyps may be limited to the superficial one-third, or even just the surface of the mucosa. As the name implies, the mucin in this type of polyp is strictly of goblet-cell type. Mucin-poor hyperplastic polyps are the least common variant encountered. Goblet cells are decreased or absent in this type of polyp, and they may show prominent nuclear atypia.

Traditional Serrated Adenoma

As previously described, the term serrated adenoma was originally applied to a subset of polyps that had a serrated hyperplasticlike architecture and adenomatous changes or dysplasia.[3] In the original report, serrated adenomas made up less than 1% of all colorectal polyps. More recent studies, however, report a higher incidence, most likely because of the wider acceptance and recognition of these lesions. In a recent review from Finland, 15.9% of colorectal polyps were diagnosed as serrated adenoma.[16] Other studies have shown that traditional serrated adenoma is identified in up to 7% of colonoscopies, with most polyps (54%) occurring on the left side of the colon.[3,13] Traditional serrated adenomas often have a pedunculated or broad-based polypoid pattern of growth, with a cerebriform or flower petal-like endoscopic appearance.[12,17–19] Small polyps, however, are endoscopically indistinguishable from hyperplastic polyps.[13]

Traditional serrated adenomas, as defined by Longacre and Fenoglio-Preiser,[3] are distinguished from sessile serrated adenomas (see later discussion) because they are comprised of a uniform population of abnormal epithelial cells with a characteristic histologic appearance. These cells are tall and columnar with brightly eosinophilic cytoplasm and a centrally placed, elongated, hyperchromatic nucleus (**Fig. 2**). Some degree of nuclear pseudostratification is typically present, but not to the same extent seen in a typical tubular or villous adenoma. Traditional serrated adenomas also commonly show the presence of so-called ectopic crypts (**Fig. 3**) in which the normal relationship of the crypts with the adjacent muscularis mucosae is no longer preserved.[11] Ectopic crypts appear shortened, and do not contact the muscularis mucosae as do normal colonic crypts. Ki-67 immunostains localize the proliferative compartment of the mucosa to these ectopic crypts, a finding that is distinctly different from that observed in traditional adenomas or hyperplastic polyps (see **Fig. 3**). Cytokeratin 20 staining is limited for the most part to the surface epithelium in this type of polyp.[11]

Sessile Serrated Adenoma

Torlakovic and Snover[9] recognized in 1996 that the hyperplastic polyps seen in association with hyperplastic polyposis differed morphologically from traditional hyperplastic polyps. These polyps have been subsequently termed sessile serrated adenomas. They have a tendency to be right-sided, large, and endoscopically flat and poorly circumscribed, sometimes mimicking enlarged folds.[11] In 1 study, sessile serrated adenomas made up 9% of all colorectal polyps, and 22% of serrated polyps in patients undergoing screening colonoscopy.[20] The histologic diagnosis of sessile serrated adenoma is based mainly on the architectural features of the lesion, which include branched crypts, dilation of the bases of the crypts, and formation of inverted L- or T-shaped crypts (**Fig. 4**). The cells lining the crypts appear mature with a goblet cell or gastric foveolar cell phenotype. Serration is often not limited to the upper portion of the crypt as is seen in typical hyperplastic polyps, but extends downward all the way to the crypt base. Focal surface nuclear pseudostratification and

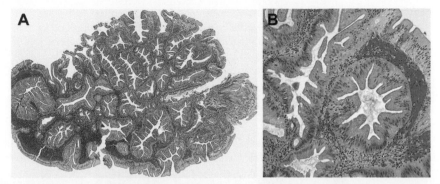

Fig. 2. Traditional serrated adenoma. (*A*) Low-power photomicrograph showing a polypoid lesion made up of glands with brightly eosinophilic cytoplasm. (*B*) Higher-power view showing the prominent serration of the colonic crypts. The cells lining the crypts are tall and columnar with eosinophilic cytoplasm. The nuclei are mildly enlarged and appear somewhat stratified.

eosinophilic change similar to that seen in traditional serrated adenoma is sometimes observed focally. Minor nuclear changes including irregular nuclear contours, an open chromatin pattern, and small prominent nucleoli may also be present. The normal pattern of cell proliferation and cytokeratin 20 staining is disturbed in sessile serrated adenomas, with Ki-67 staining irregularly along the length of the crypt, and often asymmetrically within individual crypts.[15]

Mixed Polyps

There is considerable overlap among the histologic features of hyperplastic polyps, sessile serrated adenomas, and traditional serrated adenomas, and some polyps may contain components resembling several types of serrated polyp. In large sessile serrated adenomas, for example, one often finds areas with histologic features typical

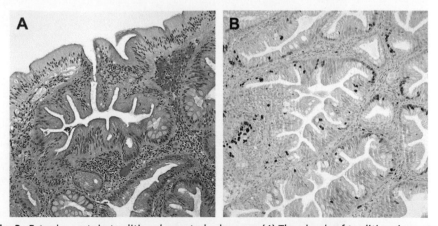

Fig. 3. Ectopic crypts in traditional serrated adenoma. (*A*) The glands of traditional serrated adenomas show small outpouchings termed ectopic crypts. (*B*) Mib-1 (Ki-67) immunostained section showing a shift in the normal proliferative zone from the base of the true colonic crypt to the bases of the ectopic crypts.

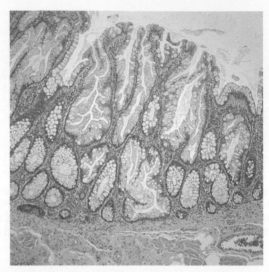

Fig. 4. Sessile serrated adenoma. Low-power view showing the architecture of a sessile serrated adenoma. The crypts are somewhat dilated, and the serration of the lumen extends to the crypt base. There is focal lateral extension of the crypt to form an inverted T-shape.

of a hyperplastic polyp. This is usually only a focal phenomenon, and classification of the polyp as sessile serrated adenoma is not difficult. Sessile serrated adenomas may also show focal areas with eosinophilic cellular changes resembling those of traditional serrated adenoma (**Fig. 5**). Similarly, some sessile serrated adenomas or traditional serrated adenomas contain areas of typical tubular or tubulovillous adenoma. This form of mixed polyp is more common than the mixed sessile serrated adenoma-traditional serrated adenoma.[21] It is likely that the transition from sessile serrated

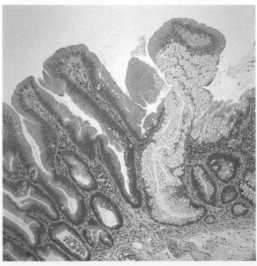

Fig. 5. This polyp shows features of sessile serrated adenoma (*right*) and traditional serrated adenoma (*left*).

adenoma to traditional adenoma represents a progression of sessile serrated adenoma to a more aggressive form of polyp because sessile serrated adenomas associated with carcinoma often show foci of typical adenoma adjacent to the invading adenocarcinoma.

Hyperplastic Polyposis

Hyperplastic polyposis is a rare syndrome that was first described in 1980 as meta-plastic polyposis.[22] Numerous reports of patients with hyperplastic polyposis associated with the development of colorectal carcinoma now exist in the literature,[5,7,23–32] suggesting that patients with this syndrome are at increased risk for developing colon cancer. Some studies suggest that colorectal cancer risk in patients with hyperplastic polyposis may be as high as 50%; patients may present with multiple synchronous or metachronous cancers.[7,24,31,33–38] Familial aggregation of the disorder has been observed in some patients, but a definite genetic association has not been established.[7,25,39] The diagnostic criteria for hyperplastic polyposis suggested by the World Health Organization are listed in **Box 2**.[40]

Patients with hyperplastic polyposis, in particular those who also develop colorectal cancer, have polyps of varying histology, with some representing typical hyperplastic polyps, others sessile serrated adenomas, traditional serrated adenomas, or classic tubular or villous adenomas.

MOLECULAR BIOLOGIC CHANGES
Adenoma and Colorectal Carcinoma

The role of the traditional adenoma in colorectal cancer development was clearly established when Vogelstein and colleagues[41] published their seminal paper reporting that a stepwise accumulation of molecular alterations accompanies the colorectal adenoma-carcinoma sequence. The earliest molecular abnormality identified in this pathway was mutation in *APC*, the gene known to be involved in familial adenomatous polyposis coli. *APC* mutation was followed by acquisition of mutations in *KRAS* and *P53* in increasingly large adenomas and invasive cancer. The adenoma-carcinoma molecular pathway applies predominantly to sporadic colorectal cancers but also characterizes familial adenomatous polyposis and is thus sometimes called the adenomatous polyposis coli (APC) pathway. Alternatively, this pathway may be referred to as the chromosomal instability pathway because colorectal tumors arising by this pathway are characterized by gross chromosomal abnormalities including deletions, insertions, and loss of heterozygosity.

Subsequently, another molecular pathway leading from adenomatous polyps to colorectal cancer (the DNA mismatch repair pathway) was described.[42] The DNA mismatch repair pathway is operative in colorectal cancers arising in association with hereditary nonpolyposis colon cancer (HNPCC) or Lynch syndrome. The key

---

Box 2
Diagnostic criteria for hyperplastic polyposis

1. At least 5 histologically confirmed hyperplastic (serrated) polyps proximal to the sigmoid colon, of which 2 are greater than 1 cm in diameter

2. Any number of hyperplastic (serrated) polyps proximal to the sigmoid colon in a subject with a first-degree relative with hyperplastic polyposis

3. More than 30 hyperplastic (serrated) polyps of any size distributed evenly throughout the colon.

element of this pathway is dysfunctional DNA mismatch repair,[43] which results from germline mutations in 1 of several DNA mismatch repair genes, most commonly *MLH1* or *MSH2*. The loss of DNA mismatch repair function results in accumulation of mutations, most commonly in repetitive microsatellite regions of the genome.[44] The result is the development of microsatellite instability (MSI) in the tumors that arise through this pathway. Genes containing such microsatellite repeat sequences are frequently altered in HNPCC, and include transforming growth factor β receptor II, insulinlike growth factor receptor 2, and Bax,[45–47] among others. Tumors arising via the DNA mismatch repair pathway characteristically have a diploid DNA content, and fail to show evidence of chromosomal losses or gains as is commonly seen in cancers arising via the APC pathway.[48,49]

Abnormalities in mismatch repair do not occur only in colorectal cancers associated with HNPCC, but are identifiable in approximately 15% of sporadic colorectal adenocarcinomas. The molecular mechanism by which these sporadic tumors develop, however, seems to be different from that of the syndromic mismatch repair deficient tumors. Sporadic adenomas rarely show high levels of MSI (MSI-H), and those that are MSI positive almost always turn out to be HNPCC associated. In addition, the early molecular alterations typically found in small adenomatous polyps such as APC loss or KRAS mutations are unusual in sporadic microsatellite unstable colorectal cancers.[50–52] In addition, alterations in other components of the wnt signaling pathway such as β-catenin[51,53] do not seem to play a role in these cancers. Other wnt signaling components such as AXIN2[54] or TCF4[55] are sometimes altered in sporadic MSI-H cancers. These alterations, however, likely do not represent surrogate markers for APC inactivation because they occur following the acquisition of MSI rather than early in tumor development. These findings suggest that nonhereditary MSI-H colorectal cancers arise by a different mechanism or mechanisms than the MSI-H cancers that characterize HNPCC.

Serrated Neoplasia Pathway

Triggered by the morphologic observations, molecular studies now provide convincing evidence that a molecular pathway (or pathways) from serrated polyps (sessile serrated adenoma and traditional serrated adenoma) to colorectal carcinoma exists. Different genetic alterations than those traditionally seen in the adenoma-carcinoma sequence have clearly been shown in serrated polyps and serrated carcinomas.[56–59] For example, APC and TP53 mutations and loss of heterozygosity are uncommon in serrated polyps, whereas alterations in microsatellite sequences and hypermethylation of CpG islands are commonly found.

Molecular studies of serrated polyps and their associated adenocarcinomas also show that there are likely 2 categories of serrated lesion that evolve by separate, but somewhat overlapping, pathways. The first consists of cancers arising predominantly in the right colon that show high levels of MSI and CpG island methylation. The precursor for these cancers is likely the sessile serrated adenoma. The second comprises tumors arising mainly in the left colon that are characteristically microsatellite stable (MSS) or MSI-L and are associated with mutations in *KRAS*.[60] This type of cancer is likely preceded by the polypoid, traditional serrated adenoma.

MAPK-ERK PATHWAY ALTERATIONS
KRAS Mutation

K-ras and B-raf are components of the MAPK-ERK pathway that mediates cellular responses to many extracellular signals regulating programmed cell death, growth, and differentiation. The *KRAS* gene encodes a 21-kDa guanosine triphosphate protein, p21^{ras}, that mediates signaling events regulating cell proliferation. Mutation results in continuous activation of the gene and leads to autonomous uncontrolled cell proliferation.

KRAS mutations are encountered in approximately one-quarter of traditional colorectal adenomas,[61–63] and are present in 40% of colorectal carcinomas overall.[64–66] Overall, *KRAS* mutations occur in from 4% to 37% of serrated polyps.[56,61–63,67–71] Before the recognition of the existence of sessile serrated adenomas, conflicting reports of the incidence of KRAS mutations in serrated adenoma appeared in the literature, most likely as a result of variability in the morphologic definitions of these lesions. However, since the development of better-defined morphologic criteria separating serrated lesions, it has become clear that KRAS mutations occur in approximately 80% of serrated rectal lesions and traditional serrated adenomas, and are rare in sessile serrated adenomas (0%–10%) that occur predominantly in the right colon.[61–63,69,70,72]

Thirty-seven percent of typical hyperplastic polyps show mutations in *KRAS*,[73] a number similar to that observed in nonserrated adenomatous polyps. *KRAS* mutations are most commonly observed in the goblet cell type of hyperplastic polyp, occurring in 43%.[62,63] In contrast, *KRAS* mutations are found in only 13% to 19% of microvesicular hyperplastic polyps.[62,63,73]

BRAF Mutation

B-raf, like K-ras, is a member of the RAF family of serine/threonine kinases, and represents a component of the RAS/RAF/MAP-kinase pathway. Activated B-raf promotes cell proliferation and in addition plays an antiapoptotic role in the cell. *BRAF* knockout mice die in utero as a result of increased apoptosis in differentiated endothelial cells,[74] and B-raf overexpression inactivates caspases, thereby inhibiting apoptosis.[75] The most common *BRAF* mutation in human tumors is a T to A transversion at nucleotide 1796 that results in a V599E amino acid substitution. This alteration mimics phosphorylation of the protein, resulting in its constitutive activation.[75,76] *BRAF* activating mutations occur in a large percentage of melanomas, and in from 5% to 15% of colorectal cancers.[76–78] When *BRAF* mutations occur in colorectal cancers, they are strongly associated with MSI and DNA methylation abnormalities.[68,70,76–79] However, *BRAF* mutations do not occur in MSI-H colorectal cancers arising in patients with HNPCC, a finding that strengthens the argument that sporadic and hereditary MSI-H cancers differ biologically.[80]

BRAF mutations are rare in adenomatous polyps, hyperplastic aberrant crypt foci, and typical hyperplastic polyps,[20,61,81] but are common in other serrated lesions. *BRAF* mutations are found in 75% to 82% of sessile serrated adenomas, 40% to 89% of mixed serrated and adenomatous polyps, and in polyps derived from patients with hyperplastic polyposis.[61,81,82] Traditional serrated adenomas show less frequent *BRAF* mutation, with approximately 20% to 33% being affected.[61,68,70]

Mutations in *KRAS* and *BRAF* in serrated polyps are mutually exclusive.[20,70,77]

EPHB2 Alterations

EphB2 is a member of a large family of receptor tyrosine kinases. Eph receptors are transmembrane proteins important in determining the spatial organization of several cell types in a variety of tissues. In intestinal epithelial cells, EphB2 and EphBe direct cell differentiation along the crypt-villus axis by downregulating the MAPK-ERK pathway via Ras and Raf.[83,84] EphB2 down-regulation results in sustained activation of the MAPK-ERK pathway in a manner analogous to the activation of Ras or Raf. The gene encoding EphB2 is located at 1p36, a locus that is lost in 13% of serrated polyps arising in association with hyperplastic polyposis.[39] In addition, the *EPHB2* promoter is methylated in 63%, and loss of heterozygosity at the *EPHB2* locus occurs in 25% of serrated adenocarcinomas.[85] These alterations are accompanied by loss of expression of EphB2, a feature that can be detected by immunohistochemistry.[85] The role of *EPHB2* in sporadic serrated polyps is currently unknown.

Alterations in Regulation of Apoptosis

Inhibition of apoptosis is common in serrated colorectal lesions. It is believed that this inhibition of programmed cell death is the major factor leading to the development of the serrated crypt lining in these lesions. Decreased cell loss through apoptosis results in accumulation of cells within the crypt. These cells then become piled up, creating the characteristic serrated appearance of the epithelium.[86] As discussed earlier, inhibition of apoptotic signaling in serrated colon lesions is believed to occur as a result of activating Ras and Raf mutations.[60,65,70] The resulting inhibition of apoptosis in serrated polyps may result in increased methylation of CpG islands, because older cells frequently show increased levels of methylation. Decreased apoptotic activity coupled with increased methylation could result in progressive dysregulation of programmed cell death as other genes involved in apoptosis such as p14 and p16 are potentially methylated.[80,87] Inhibition of apoptosis is especially common in serrated adenomas compared with hyperplastic polyps or conventional adenomas.[86,88–91]

DNA Methylation Alterations

DNA methylation is an essential epigenetic mechanism regulating gene expression. It is critical in such processes as DNA imprinting, X chromosome inactivation, and control of tissue-specific gene expression.[92,93] DNA methylation commonly occurs at sites of repetitive cytosine-guanine sequences termed CpG islands. CpG dinucleotides occur in dense clusters in the promoter regions of many genes. Methylation of the cytosine residues in these clusters results in inactivation of the promoter, with resultant gene silencing. Methylation of the promoters of tumor suppressor genes represents an alternate mechanism to mutation or chromosomal loss for their inactivation.[94]

Overall, 30% to 50% of colorectal cancers show evidence of excess CpG island methylation.[63,69,70,95–99] This phenomenon has been referred to as the CpG island methylator phenotype (CIMP),[94] and may be divided into low- (CIMP-L) and high-level (CIMP-H) forms. Patients with CIMP-positive colorectal cancers are distinct from those with CIMP-negative tumors in that they are older and more likely to be female. In addition CIMP-positive tumors are more commonly right-sided, mucinous, poorly differentiated, microsatellite unstable, and harbor BRAF mutations.[70,94,100,101] CIMP-H occurs in nearly 70% of sessile serrated adenomas, 47% of microvesicular hyperplastic polyps, and only 15% of goblet cell hyperplastic polyps.[62,96] CIMP-H is more frequently identified in hyperplastic polyps from the right than from the left side of the colon.

In the serrated neoplasia pathway, CpG island methylation is an early phenomenon, occurring even in aberrant crypt foci[81] or small hyperplastic polyps.[98] CpG island methylation may also be identified in histologically normal colonic mucosa of some patients with hyperplastic polyposis[102] or colorectal cancer.[103] This finding suggests that abnormal methylation may represent the underlying abnormality in many cancers arising by way of the serrated neoplasia pathway. Genes frequently inactivated by promoter methylation in serrated colon lesions include MLH1 (associated with MSI-H), O-6-methyguanine DNA methyltransferase (MGMT) (associated with MSI-L), p14, p16, and EphB2 (associated with inhibition of apoptosis).[62,63,80,85,87,104–109] The result of this variable inactivation of target genes is that CIMP-positive colorectal cancers are not a homogeneous group, but instead comprise 2 major subgroups: 1 that is MSI-H, and a second that is MSI-L or MSS.[100]

The mechanism by which CIMP-H occurs is unknown, but there is a strong association between tumors that show *BRAF* mutations and are CIMP-H and a positive family history for colorectal cancer.[110–112] A genetic predisposition to DNA methylation may also exist among patients with hyperplastic polyposis. One study found extensive DNA methylation in the normal colonic mucosa from 3 patients with hyperplastic polyposis.[102] In addition, some patients with hyperplastic polyposis develop multiple colorectal cancers, of which some are MSS, and others MSI-L or MSI-H.[35] This finding could be explained by an underlying predisposition to CpG island methylation, which leads to differing methylation patterns in different tumors in the same patient.

MSI and DNA Mismatch Repair Abnormalities

As discussed previously, MSI was first described in tumors arising in patients with HNPCC. In more than 90% of these patients, inherited mutations in DNA mismatch repair genes, most commonly MLH1 and MSH2 but also rarely MSH6 and PMS2, lead to MSI-H cancers.[42,113–115] In sporadic colon cancers, MSI-H almost always results from loss of MLH1 function, which occurs as a result of promoter methylation rather than gene mutation.[105,116] Methylation of other DNA mismatch repair genes is rare in sporadic MSI-H tumors.

MLH1 methylation has been detected in 36% of hyperplastic polyps, 70% of sessile serrated adenomas, and almost 90% of sporadic MSI-H colorectal cancers.[80,105,117] Loss of MLH1 expression as determined by immunohistochemistry has also been reported in sessile serrated adenomas and mixed polyps, but generally does not occur in hyperplastic polyps and traditional serrated adenomas.[58,73,104,118] This finding suggests that sessile serrated adenomas likely represent the precursor lesion for MSI-H sporadic colon cancers. *KRAS* mutations are infrequent in MSI-H colorectal cancers, but *BRAF* mutations are common.[39,50,51,56,70]

MGMT Alterations

A subset of colorectal carcinomas shows evidence of low-level MSI. The significance of the MSI-L phenotype is controversial, and although the colorectal carcinomas with MSI-L do not form a well-defined group, there is evidence to suggest that MSI-L is a nonrandom phenomenon with a biologic basis.[119,120] MSI-L colorectal cancer is not associated with silencing of MLH1 or any of the other known DNA mismatch repair genes.[85,119,121] The MSI-L phenotype has been associated with methylation of the promoter for the DNA repair gene MGMT. It has been hypothesized that deficient expression of MGMT results in accumulation of methylG:T mismatches and excess stress on the mismatch repair system, leading ultimately to MSI-L.[87,106,117]

MGMT methylation is rare in HNPCC, occurring in approximately 6% of tumors from this group of patients.[80] In contrast, MGMT methylation or loss of MGMT expression occurs in 14% to 22% of hyperplastic polyps,[61,63] 23% to 25% of sessile serrated adenomas,[61,63] and 16% to 78% of serrated adenomas that harbor some degree of dysplasia.[61,87] Fifty percent of serrated adenocarcinomas show evidence of MGMT promoter methylation,[87] and almost 30% are MSI-L.[122] In contrast, the MSI-L phenotype is observed in only 13.7% of nonserrated colorectal carcinomas.[122] This finding favors the idea that factors leading to MSI-L may be important in the serrated neoplasia pathway. MGMT and MLH1 methylation may coexist in MSI-H colorectal cancers, most likely resulting from high levels of CpG island methylation.[80]

The Serrated Neoplasia Pathway

Based on molecular studies, 5 molecular subtypes of colorectal cancer likely exist[123] (**Table 1**). In the first 2 subtypes, colon cancers arise in preexisting adenomas. In 1 of these groups, tumors display chromosomal instability, and are mainly MSS and CIMP negative. These tumors follow the traditional APC or chromosomal instability pathway and may be inherited (familial adenomatous polyposis or *MUTYH* polyposis) or sporadic. The second group includes those tumors arising in association with HNPCC. These tumors are CIMP-negative, MSI-H, chromosomally stable, and do not show mutation in *BRAF*.

Two additional subgroups arise from serrated polyps. The first group comprises 12% of colorectal cancers. They are CIMP-H, MSI-H, show BRAF mutation, and are chromosomally stable.[123] These tumors most likely arise from preexisting sessile serrated adenomas located in the right colon. Second are colorectal cancers that are CIMP-H, chromosomally stable, and show MGMT methylation or partial methylation of MLH1, BRAF mutation, and are MSI-L or MSS. These tumors comprise 8% of cancers, and probably arise from preexisting, left-sided, traditional serrated adenomas. Based on these observations, it is likely that 2 distinct serrated pathways exist, 1 in which cancers derive from traditional serrated adenomas, and the other in which cancers arise from sessile serrated adenomas.[124] The underlying abnormality in both pathways, however, is the same, the CIMP.

The final group of colorectal cancers is made up of tumors that are CIMP-L, chromosomally unstable, show MGMT methylation and KRAS mutation, and are MSI-L or MSS. These make up 20% of colorectal cancers. Such tumors may arise in either preexisting adenomas or serrated polyps with *KRAS* mutations. This group of tumors probably arises through what is essentially a fusion of the serrated and chromosomal instability pathways.[123]

Clinical Implications of Serrated Polyps

It is now well established that patients with traditional and sessile serrated adenomas are at increased risk for the development of colorectal cancer. The magnitude of the neoplastic risk associated with these lesions, however, is still unknown. Determination of the true frequency of hyperplastic polyps, serrated adenomas, and sessile serrated adenomas is important because it allows estimation of the true rate of malignant conversion of these lesions. In 1 study, residual serrated polyp was observed adjacent to 5.8% of colorectal cancers.[125] This is probably an underestimate of the true incidence of colorectal cancer originating in serrated polyps because most tumors outgrow and destroy the original precursor lesion. Some studies suggest that as many as 20% of colorectal cancers overall show widespread defects in DNA methylation, and that many (if not all) of these may arise within serrated polyps.[101] Combining the various types of serrated polyp with malignant potential, it is likely that the rate of conversion to malignancy is at least as great as that observed for adenomas.

Some studies suggest that the rate of progression to malignancy may be higher for serrated adenomas than for traditional colorectal adenomas.[126,127] In 1 study,[16] patients with sessile serrated adenomas developed subsequent adenomas following complete removal of the index polyp at almost twice the rate of patients with similarly treated conventional adenomas. The estimated growth rate of sessile serrated adenomas in this study was 3.76 mm/y compared with a mean of 2.79 mm/y in conventional adenomas and 1.36 mm/y in hyperplastic polyps. Patients with sessile serrated adenomas had a 5.3% rate of

Table 1
Molecular classification of colorectal carcinoma

	Chromosomal Instability Pathway	Mismatch Repair Pathway	Serrated Pathway	Hybrid Pathway
Heredity	Hereditary and sporadic	Hereditary	Hereditary and sporadic	Sporadic
CIMP status	Negative	Negative	High	Low
MSI status	MSS	MSI-H	MSI-H, MSI-L	MSI-L or MSS
Chromosomal instability	Present	Absent	Absent	Present
KRAS mutation	Common	Sometimes	Absent	Common
BRAF mutation	Absent	Absent	Common	Absent
MLH1 status	Normal	Mutation	Methylated	Partial methylation
MGMT methylation	Absent	Absent	Sometimes	Common

developing subsequent adenocarcinoma compared with a 2.2% rate in those with conventional adenomas. These observations are supported by case reports that have also documented rapid recurrence of serrated adenomas, or their rapid progression to adenocarcinoma.[128,129]

Based on these findings, most typical small hyperplastic polyps are probably innocuous lesions without significant risk for progression to more advanced lesions. Serrated adenomas, on the other hand, likely carry a significant risk for recurrence or progression. As a result, any serrated lesion larger than 1 cm should probably be completely excised and followed up endoscopically to ensure that it has not recurred. Similarly, mixed polyps containing foci of dysplasia or adenoma should be treated in a manner analogous to traditional adenomas.[130] Whether the follow-up interval for patients with serrated adenomas should be shorter than that for patients with traditional adenomas is as yet unestablished.

REFERENCES

1. Goldman H, Ming S, Hickock DF. Nature and significance of hyperplastic polyps of the human colon. Arch Pathol 1970;89(4):349–54.
2. Eide TJ. Prevalence and morphological features of adenomas of the large intestine in individuals with and without colorectal carcinoma. Histopathology 1986; 10(2):111–8.
3. Longacre TA, Fenoglio-Preiser CF. Mixed hyperplastic adenomatous polyps/ serrated adenomas. A distinct form of colorectal neoplasia. Am J Surg Pathol 1990;14(6):524–37.
4. Azimuddin K, Stasik JJ, Khubchandani IT, et al. Hyperplastic polyps: "more than meets the eye"? Report of sixteen cases. Dis Colon Rectum 2000;43(9): 1309–13.
5. Warner AS, Glick ME, Fogt F. Multiple large hyperplastic polyps of the colon coincident with adenocarcinoma. Am J Gastroenterol 1994;89(1):123–5.
6. Urbanski SJ, Kossakowska AE, Marcon N, et al. Mixed hyperplastic adenomatous polyps: an underdiagnosed entity; report of a case of adenocarcinoma arising within a mixed hyperplastic adenomatous polyp. Am J Surg Pathol 1984;8(7):551–6.
7. Jeevaratnam P, Cottier DS, Browett PJ, et al. Familial giant hyperplastic polyposis predisposing to colorectal cancer: a new hereditary bowel cancer syndrome. J Pathol 1996;179(1):20–5.
8. Renaut AJ, Douglas PR, Newstead GL. Hyperplastic polyposis of the colon and rectum. Colorectal Dis 2002;4(3):213–5.
9. Torlakovic E, Snover DC. Serrated adenomatous polyposis in humans. Gastroenterology 1996;110(3):748–55.
10. Torlakovic E, Skovlund E, Snover DC, et al. Morphologic reappraisal of serrated colorectal polyps. Am J Surg Pathol 2003;27(1):65–81.
11. DiSario JA, Foutch PG, Mai HD, et al. Prevalence and malignant potential of colorectal polyps in asymptomatic, average-risk men. Am J Gastroenterol 1991;86(8):941–5.
12. Oka S, Tanaka S, Hiyama T, et al. Clinicopathologic and endoscopic features of colorectal serrated adenoma: differences between polypoid and superficial types. Gastrointest Endosc 2004;59(2):213–9.
13. Jamarillo E, Tamura S, Mitomi H. Endoscopic appearance of serrated adenomas of the colon. Endoscopy 2005;37(3):254–60.

14. Higuchi T, Sugihara K, Jass JR. Demographic and pathological characteristics of serrated polyps of the colorectum. Histopathology 2005;47(1):32–40.

15. Torlakovic EE, Gomez JD, Driman DK, et al. Sessile serrated adenoma (SSA) vs. traditional serrated adenoma (TSA). Am J Surg Pathol 2008; 32(3):21–9.

16. Lazarus R, Junttila OE, Karttunen TJ, et al. The risk of metachronous neoplasia in patients with serrated adenoma. Am J Clin Pathol 2005;123(3): 349–59.

17. Matsumoto T, Mizuno M, Shimizu M, et al. Clinicopathologic features of serrated adenoma of the colorectum: comparison with traditional adenoma. J Clin Pathol 1999;52(7):513–6.

18. Matsumoto T, Mizuno M, Shimizu M, et al. Serrated adenoma of the colorectum: colonoscopic and histologic features. Gastrointest Endosc 1999;49(6):736–42.

19. Lee SK, Chang HJ, Kim TI, et al. Clinicopathologic findings of colorectal traditional and sessile serrated adenomas in Korea: a multicenter study. Digestion 2008;77(3–4):178–83.

20. Spring KJ, Zhao ZZ, Karamatic R, et al. High prevalence of sessile serrated adenomas with BRAF mutations: a prospective study of patients undergoing colonoscopy. Gastroenterology 2006;131(5):1400–7.

21. Snover DC, Jass JR, Fenoglio-Preiser C, et al. Serrated polyps of the large intestine. A morphologic and molecular review of an evolving concept. Am J Clin Pathol 2005;124(3):380–91.

22. Williams GT, Arthur JF, Bussey HJ, et al. Metaplastic polyps and polyposis of the colorectum. Histopathology 1980;4(2):155–70.

23. Abeyasundara H, Hampshire P. Hyperplastic polyposis associated with synchronous adenocarcinomas of the transverse colon. ANZ J Surg 2002; 71(11):686–7.

24. Bengoechea O, Martinez-Penuela JM, Larringa B, et al. Hyperplastic polyposis of the colorectum and adenocarcinoma in a 24-year-old man. Am J Surg Pathol 1987;11(4):323–7.

25. Ferrandez A, Samowitz W, DiSario JA, et al. Phenotypic characteristics and risk of cancer development in hyperplastic polyposis: case series and literature review. Am J Gastroenterol 2004;99(10):2012–8.

26. Jorgensen H, Mogensen AM, Svendsen LB. Hyperplastic polyposis of the large bowel. Three cases and a review of the literature. Scand J Gastroenterol 1996; 31(8):825–30.

27. Keljo DJ, Weinberg AG, Winick N, et al. Rectal cancer in an 11-year-old girl with hyperplastic polyposis. J Pediatr Gastroenterol Nutr 1998;28(3):327–32.

28. Koide N, Saito Y, Fujii T, et al. A case of hyperplastic polyposis of the colon with adenocarcinomas in hyperplastic polyps after long-term follow-up. Endoscopy 2002;34(6):499–502.

29. Leggett BA, Devereaux B, Biden K, et al. Hyperplastic polyposis: association with colorectal cancer. Am J Surg Pathol 2001;25(2):177–84.

30. Lieverse RJ, Kibbelaar RE, Griffioen G, et al. Colonic adenocarcinoma in a patient with multiple hyperplastic polyps. Neth J Med 1995;46(4):185–8.

31. McCann BG. A case of metaplastic polyposis of the colon associated with focal adenomatous change and metachronous adenocarcinomas. Histopathology 1998;13(6):700–2.

32. Orii S, Nakamura S, Sugai T, et al. Hyperplastic (metaplastic) polyposis of the colorectum associated with adenomas and an adenocarcinoma. J Clin Gastroenterol 1997;25(1):369–72.

33. Shepherd NA. Inverted hyperplastic polyposis of the colon. J Clin Pathol 1993; 46(1):56–60.
34. Teoh HH, Delahunt B, Isbister WH. Dysplastic and malignant areas in hyperplastic polyps of the large intestine. Pathology 1989;21(2):138–42.
35. Jass JR, Iino H, Ruszkiewicz A, et al. Neoplastic progression occurs through mutator pathways in hyperplastic polyposis of the colorectum. Gut 2000; 47(1):43–9.
36. Yao T, Nishiyama K, Oya M, et al. Multiple 'serrated adenocarcinomas' of the colon with a cell lineage common to metaplastic polyps and serrated adenoma: case report of a new subtype of colonic adenocarcinoma with gastric differentiation. J Pathol 2000;190(4):444–9.
37. Chow E, Lipton L, Lynch E, et al. Hyperplastic polyposis syndrome: phenotypic presentations and the role of MBD4 and MYH. Gastroenterology 2006;131(1):30–9.
38. Hyman NH, Anderson P, Blasyk H. Hyperplastic polyposis and the risk of colorectal cancer. Dis Colon Rectum 2004;47(12):2101–4.
39. Rashid A, Houlihan PS, Booker S, et al. Phenotypic and molecular characteristics of hyperplastic polyposis. Gastroenterology 2000;119(2):323–32.
40. Burt R, Jass JR. Hyperplastic polyposis. In: Hamilton SR, Aaltonen LA, editors, Pathology and genetics of tumours of the digestive system: World Health Organization Classification of Tumours, vol 2. Lyon: IARC; 2000. p. 135–6.
41. Vogelstein B, Fearon ER, Hamilton SR, et al. Genetic alterations during colorectal tumor development. N Engl J Med 1988;319(9):525–32.
42. Aaltonen LA, Peltomaki P, Leach FS, et al. Clues to the pathogenesis of familial colorectal cancer. Science 1993;260(5109):812–6.
43. Thibodeau SN, French AJ, Roche PC, et al. Altered expression of hMSH2 and hMLH1 in tumors with microsatellite instability and genetic alterations in mismatch repair genes. Cancer Res 1996;56(21):4836–40.
44. Iino H, Simms L, Young J, et al. DNA microsatellite instability and mismatch repair protein loss in adenomas presenting in hereditary non-polyposis colorectal cancer. Gut 2000;47(1):37–42.
45. Markowitz S, Wang J, Myeroff L, et al. Inactivation of the type II TGF-β receptor in colon cancer cells with microsatellite instability. Science 1995;268(5215): 1336–8.
46. Rampino N, Yamamoto H, Ionov Y, et al. Somatic frameshift mutations in the BAX gene in colon cancers of the microsatellite mutator phenotype. Science 1997; 275(5302):967–9.
47. Souza RF, Appel R, Yin J, et al. Microsatellite instability in the insulin-like growth factor II receptor gene in gastrointestinal tumours. Nat Genet 1996;14(3):225–7.
48. Ionov Y, Peinado MA, Malkhosyan S, et al. Ubiquitous somatic mutations in simple repeated sequences reveal a new mechanism for colonic carcinogenesis. Nature 1993;363(6429):558–61.
49. Kinzler KW, Vogelstein B. Lessons from hereditary colorectal cancer. Cell 1996; 87(2):159–70.
50. Salahshor S, Kressner U, Pahlman L, et al. Colorectal cancer with and without microsatellite instability involves different genes. Genes Chromosomes Cancer 1999;26(3):247–52.
51. Jass JR, Biden KG, Cummings M, et al. Characterisation of a subtype of colorectal cancer combining features of the suppressor and mild mutator pathways. J Clin Pathol 1999;52(6):455–60.

52. Jass JR, Barker M, Fraser L, et al. APC mutation and tumour budding in colorectal cancer. J Clin Pathol 2003;56(1):69–73.
53. Wong NA, Morris RG, McCondochie A, et al. Cyclin D1 overexpression in colorectal carcinoma in vivo is dependent on β-catenin protein dysregulation, but not k-ras mutation. J Pathol 2002;197(1):128–35.
54. Liu W, Dong X, Mai M, et al. Mutations in AXIN2 cause colorectal cancer with defective mismatch repair by activating beta-catenin/TCF signaling. Nat Genet 2000;26(2):146–7.
55. Thorstensen L, Lind GE, Lovig T, et al. Genetic and epigenetic changes of components affecting the WNT pathway in colorectal carcinomas stratified by microsatellite instability. Neoplasia 2005;7(2):99–108.
56. Ajioka Y, Watanabe H, Jass JR, et al. Infrequent K-ras codon 12 mutation in serrated adenomas of human colorectum. Gut 1998;42(5):680–4.
57. Uchida H, Ando H, Maruyama K, et al. Genetic alterations of mixed hyperplastic adenomatous polyps in the colon and rectum. Jpn J Cancer Res 1998;89(3): 299–306.
58. Sawyer EJ, Cerar A, Hanby AM, et al. Molecular characteristics of serrated adenomas. Gut 2002;51(2):200–6.
59. Yamamoto T, Konishi K, Yamochi T, et al. No major tumorigenic role for beta-catenin in serrated as opposed to conventional colorectal adenomas. Br J Cancer 2003;89(1):152–7.
60. Jass JR, Whitehall VL, Young J, et al. Emerging concepts in colorectal neoplasia. Gastroenterology 2002;123(3):862–76.
61. Jass JR, Baker K, Zlobec I, et al. Advanced colorectal polyps with the molecular and morphological features of serrated polyps and adenomas: concept of a 'fusion' pathway to colorectal cancer. Histopathology 2006; 49(2):121–31.
62. O'Brien MJ, Yang S, Clebanoff JL, et al. Hyperplastic (serrated) polyps of the colorectum. Relationship of CpG island methylator phenotype and K-ras mutation to location and histologic subtype. Am J Surg Pathol 2004;28(4):423–34.
63. O'Brien MJ, Yang S, Mack C, et al. Comparison of microsatellite instability, CpG island methylation phenotype, BRAF and KRAS status in serrated polyps and traditional adenomas indicates separate pathways to distinct colorectal carcinoma end points. Am J Surg Pathol 2006;30(12):1491–501.
64. Barry EL, Baron JA, Grau MV, et al. K-ras mutation in incident sporadic colorectal adenomas. Cancer 2006;106(5):1036–40.
65. Guerrero S, Casanova I, Farre L, et al. K-ras codon 12 mutations induces higher level of resistance to apoptosis and predisposition to anchorage-independent growth than codon 13 mutation or proto-oncogene overexpression. Cancer Res 2000;60(23):6750–6.
66. Maltzman T, Knoll K, Martinez ME, et al. Ki-ras proto-oncogene mutations in sporadic colorectal adenomas: relationship to histologic and clinical characteristics. Gastroenterology 2001;121(2):302–9.
67. Otori K, Oda Y, Sugiyama K, et al. High frequency of K-ras mutations in human colorectal hyperplastic polyps. Gut 1997;40(5):660–3.
68. Chan TL, Zhao W, Leung SY, et al. BRAF and KRAS mutations in colorectal hyperplastic polyps and serrated adenomas. Cancer Res 2003;63(16): 4878–81.
69. Yang S, Farraye FA, Mack C, et al. BRAF and KRAS mutations in hyperplastic polyps and serrated adenomas of the colorectum: relationship to histology and CpG island methylation status. Am J Surg Pathol 2004;28(11):1452–9.

70. Kambara T, Simms L, Whitehall VL, et al. BRAF mutation and CpG island methylation: an alternative pathway to colorectal cancer. Gut 2004;53(8): 1137–44.
71. Zauber P, Sabbath-Solitare M, Marotta S, et al. Comparative molecular pathology of sporadic hyperplastic polyps and neoplastic lesions from the same individual. J Clin Pathol 2004;57(10):1084–8.
72. Higashidani Y, Tamura S, Morita T, et al. Analysis of K-ras codon 12 mutation in flat and nodular variants of serrated adenoma in the colon. Dis Colon Rectum 2003;46(3):327–32.
73. Yashiro M, Laghi L, Saito K, et al. Serrated adenomas have a pattern of genetic alterations that distinguishes them from other colorectal polyps. Cancer Epidemiol Biomarkers Prev 2005;14(9):2253–6.
74. Baccarini M. An old kinase on a new path: Raf and apoptosis. Cell Death Differ 2002;9(8):783–5.
75. Mercer KE, Pritchard CA. Raf proteins and cancer: B-Raf is identified as a mutational target. Biochim Biophys Acta 2003;1653(1):25–40.
76. Davies H, Bignell GR, Cox C, et al. Mutations of the BRAF gene in human cancer. Nature 2002;417(6892):949–54.
77. Rajagopalan H, Bardelli A, Lengauer C, et al. Tumorigenesis: RAF/RAS oncogenes and mismatch repair status. Nature 2002;418(6901):934.
78. Yuen ST, Davies H, Chan TL, et al. Similarity of the phenotypic patterns associated with BRAF and KRAS mutations in colorectal neoplasia. Cancer Res 2002; 62(22):6451–5.
79. Weisenberger DJ, Siegmund KD, Campan M, et al. CpG island methylator phenotype underlies sporadic microsatellite instability and is tightly associated with BRAF mutation in colorectal cancer. Nat Genet 2006;38(7): 787–93.
80. McGivern A, Wynter CV, Whitehall VL, et al. Promoter hypermethylation frequency and BRAF mutations distinguish hereditary non-polyposis colon cancer syndrome from sporadic MSI-H colon cancer. Fam Cancer 2004; 3(2):101–7.
81. Beach R, Chan AO, Wu TT, et al. BRAF mutations in aberrant crypt foci and hyperplastic polyposis. Am J Pathol 2005;166(4):1069–75.
82. Konishi K, Yamochi T, Makino R, et al. Molecular differences between sporadic serrated and conventional colorectal adenomas. Clin Cancer Res 2004;10(9): 3082–90.
83. Batlle E, Henderson JT, Beghtel H, et al. Beta-catenin and TCF mediate cell positioning in the intestinal epithelium by controlling the expression of EphB/ ephrin B. Cell 2002;111(2):251–63.
84. Elowe S, Holland SJ, Kulkarni S, et al. Downregulation of the ras-mitogen-activated protein kinase pathway by the EphB2 receptor tyrosine kinase is required for ephrin-induced neurite retraction. Mol Cell Biol 2001;21(21):7429–41.
85. Laiho P, Kokko A, Vanharanta S, et al. Serrated carcinomas form a subclass of colorectal cancer with distinct molecular basis. Oncogene 2007;26(2):312–20.
86. Tateyama H, Li W, Takahashi E, et al. Apoptosis index and apoptosis-related antigen expression in serrated adenoma of the colorectum: the saw-toothed structure may be related to inhibition of apoptosis. Am J Surg Pathol 2002; 26(2):249–56.
87. Dong SM, Lee EJ, Jeon ES, et al. Progressive methylation during the serrated neoplasia pathway of the colorectum. Mod Pathol 2005;18(2):170–8.

88. Horkko TT, Makinen MJ. Colorectal proliferation and apoptosis in serrated versus conventional adenoma-carcinoma pathway: growth, progression and survival. Scand J Gastroenterol 2003;38(12):1241–8.
89. Komori K, Ajioka Y, Watanabe H, et al. Proliferation kinetics and apoptosis of serrated adenoma of the colorectum. Pathol Int 2003;53(5):277–83.
90. Ladas SD, Kitsanta P, Triantafyllou K, et al. Cell turnover of serrated adenomas. J Pathol 2005;206(1):62–7.
91. Mitomi H, Sada M, Kobayashi K, et al. Different apoptotic activity and p21$^{WAF1/CIP1}$, but not p27^{Kip1}, expression in serrated adenomas as compared with traditional adenomas and hyperplastic polyps of the colorectum. J Cancer Res Clin Oncol 2003;129(8):449–55.
92. Jubb AM, Bell SM, Quirke P. Methylation and colorectal cancer. J Pathol 2001; 195(1):111–34.
93. Robertson KD, Wolffe AP. DNA methylation in health and disease. Nat Rev Genet 2000;1(1):11–9.
94. Toyota M, Ahuja N, Ohe-Toyota M, et al. CpG island methylator phenotype in colorectal cancer. Proc Natl Acad Sci U S A 1999;96(15):8681–6.
95. Ogino S, Kawasaki T, Kirkner G, et al. Down-regulation of p21 (CDKN1A/CIP 1) is inversely associated with microsatellite instability and the CpG island methylator phenotype (CIMP) in colorectal cancer. J Pathol 2006;210(2): 147–54.
96. Park SJ, Rashid A, Lee J-H, et al. Frequent CpG island methylation in serrated adenomas of the colorectum. Am J Pathol 2003;162(3):815–22.
97. Chan AO, Issa JP, Morris JS, et al. Concordant CpG island methylation in hyperplastic polyposis. Am J Pathol 2002;160(2):529–36.
98. Kondo Y, Issa JP. Epigenetic changes in colorectal cancer. Cancer Metastasis Rev 2004;23(1–2):29–39.
99. van Rijnsoever M, Grieu F, Elsaleh H, et al. Characterisation of colorectal cancers showing hypermethylation at multiple CpG islands. Gut 2002;51(6): 797–802.
100. Whitehall VL, Wynter CV, Walsh MD, et al. Morphological and molecular heterogeneity within nonmicrosatellite instability-high colorectal cancer. Cancer Res 2002;62(21):6011–4.
101. Hawkins N, Norrie M, Cheong K, et al. CpG island methylation in sporadic colorectal cancer and its relationship to microsatellite instability. Gastroenterology 2002;122(5):1376–87.
102. Minoo P, Baker K, Goswami R, et al. Extensive DNA methylation in normal colorectal mucosa in hyperplastic polyposis. Gut 2006;55(10):1467–74.
103. Kawakami K, Ruszkiewicz A, Bennett G, et al. DNA hypermethylation in normal colonic mucosa of patients with colorectal cancer. Br J Cancer 2006;94(4): 593–8.
104. Oh K, Redston M, Odze RD. Support for hMLH1 and MGMT silencing as a mechanism of tumorigenesis in the hyperplastic-adenoma-carcinoma (serrated) carcinogenic pathway in the colon. Hum Pathol 2005;36(1):101–11.
105. Young J, Simms LA, Biden KG, et al. Features of colorectal cancers with high-level microsatellite instability occurring in familial and non-familial settings: parallel pathways of tumorigenesis. Am J Pathol 2001;159(6):2107–16.
106. Whitehall VL, Walsh MD, Young J, et al. Methylation of O-6-methylguanine-DNA methyltransferase characterizes a subset of colorectal cancer with low level DNA microsatellite instability. Cancer Res 2001;61(3):827–30.

107. Noda H, Kato Y, Yoshikawa H, et al. Microsatellite instability caused by hMHL1 promoter methylation increases with tumor progression in right-sided sporadic colorectal cancer. Oncology 2005;69(4):354–62.

108. Kuismanen SA, Holmberg MT, Salovaara R, et al. Epigenetic phenotypes distinguish microsatellite-stable and unstable colorectal cancers. Proc Natl Acad Sci U S A 1999;96(22):12661–6.

109. Kuismanen SA, Homberg MT, Salovaara R, et al. Genetic and epigenetic modification of MLH1 accounts for a major share of microsatellite-unstable colorectal cancers. Am J Pathol 2000;156(5):1773–9.

110. Samowitz WS, Sweeney C, Herrick J, et al. Poor survival associated with the BRAF V600E mutation in microsatellite stable colon cancers. Cancer Res 2005;65(14):6063–9.

111. Frazier ML, Xi L, Zong J, et al. Association of the CpG island methylator phenotype with family history of cancer in patients with colorectal cancer. Cancer Res 2003;63(16):4805–8.

112. Vandrovcova J, Lagerstedt-Robinsson K, Pahlman L, et al. Somatic BRAF V600E mutations in familial colorectal cancer. Cancer Epidemiol Biomarkers Prev 2006;15(11):2270–3.

113. Peltomaki P, Aaltonen LA, Sistonen P, et al. Genetic mapping of a locus predisposing to human colorectal cancer. Science 1993;260(5109):812–6.

114. Thibodeau SN, Bren G, Schaid D. Microsatellite instability in cancer of the proximal colon. Science 1993;260(5109):816–9.

115. Worthley DL, Walsh MD, Barker M, et al. Familial mutations in PMS2 can cause autosomal dominant hereditary nonpolyposis colorectal cancer. Gastroenterology 2005;128(5):1431–6.

116. Deng G, Bell I, Crawley S, et al. BRAF mutation is frequently present in sporadic colorectal cancer with methylated MLH1, but not in hereditary nonpolyposis colorectal cancer. Clin Cancer Res 2004;10(1 Pt 1):191–5.

117. Jass JR. Serrated adenoma of the colorectum and the DNA-methylator phenotype. Nat Clin Pract Oncol 2005;2(8):398–405.

118. Goldstein NS, Bhanot P, Odish E, et al. Hyperplastic-like colon polyps that preceded microsatellite-unstable adenocarcinomas. Am J Clin Pathol 2003; 119(6):778–96.

119. Halford S, Sasieni P, Rowan A, et al. Low-level microsatellite instability occurs in most colorectal cancers and is a nonrandomly distributed quantitative trait. Cancer Res 2002;62(1):53–7.

120. Halford SER, Sawyer EJ, Lambros MB, et al. MSI-low, a real phenomenon which varies in frequency among cancer types. J Pathol 2003;201(3):289–94.

121. Tomlinson I, Ilyas M, Johnson V, et al. A comparison of the genetic pathways involved in the pathogenesis of three types of colorectal cancer. J Pathol 1998;184(2):148–52.

122. Tuppurainen K, Makinen JM, Junttila O, et al. Morphology and microsatellite instability in sporadic serrated and non-serrated colorectal cancer. J Pathol 2005;207(3):285–94.

123. Jass JR. Classification of colorectal cancer based on correlation of clinical, morphological and molecular features. Histopathology 2007;50(1):113–30.

124. Makinen MJ. Colorectal serrated adenocarcinoma. Histopathology 2007;50(1): 131–50.

125. Makinen MJ, George SM, Jernvall P, et al. Colorectal carcinoma associated with serrated adenoma –prevalence, histological features, and prognosis. J Pathol 2001;193(3):286–94.

126. Goldstein NS. Clinical significance of (sessile) serrated adenomas: another piece of the puzzle. Am J Clin Pathol 2005;123(3):329–30.
127. Jass JR. Serrated route to colorectal cancer: back street or super highway? J Pathol 2001;193(3):283–5.
128. Yamauchi T, Watanabe M, Hasegawa H, et al. Serrated adenoma developing into advanced colon cancer in 2 years. J Gastroenterol 2002;37(6):467–70.
129. Makinen JM, Makinen MJ, Karttunen TJ. Serrated adenocarcinoma of the rectum associated with perianal Paget's disease: a case report. Histopathology 2002;41(2):177–9.
130. Cunningham KS, Riddell RH. Serrated mucosal lesions of the colorectum. Curr Opin Gastroenterol 2006;22(1):48–53.

CT Colonography and Non-Polypoid Colorectal Neoplasms

Noriko Suzuki, MD, PhD[a],*, Ana Ignjatovic, BA, BMBCh, MRCP[a],
David Burling, MD, MRCP, FRCP[b], Stuart A. Taylor, MD, MRCP, FRCP[c]

KEYWORDS

- Non-polypoid colorectal neoplasms • Flat neoplasms
- Colonography • CT colonography • Computer-assisted

Computed tomographic colonography (CTC) is a relatively new development for examining the large intestine. Some comparison with colonoscopy has suggested that CTC is as effective as optical colonoscopy in detection of significant adenomas.[1–3] However, widely conflicting performance data and critical expert commentaries have questioned whether CTC can detect flat neoplasia.[4–7] The advent of CTC, particularly when performed using the latest methods for optimizing distension and bowel preparation such as automated colonic insufflators[8] and fecal tagging,[9] provides a potentially accurate technique for detection and characterization of flat polyps.[4]

WHAT IS A FLAT POLYP?

Histologically, when the height of the polyp is more than double the thickness of adjacent mucosa, it is frequently described as a flat polyp.[10] However, this definition applies only to the operative specimen and is of no benefit to colonoscopists or radiologists. The most common endoscopic definition of a flat polyp is a polyp whose height is no more than half its diameter and this has also been used for CTC.[11] In 2000, Paris workshop participants attempted to achieve consensus for endoscopy by proposing that closed biopsy forceps (approximately 2.5 mm in height) are placed next to the polyp to estimate its height and categorize it as polypoid (>2.5 mm) or non-polypoid (<2.5 mm). More recently, a joint working party for CTC defined flat polyps as those with less than 3 mm of vertical elevation above the surrounding colonic mucosa.[12]

---

[a] Wolfson Unit for Endoscopy, St Mark's Hospital, Watford Road, Harrow, Middlesex HA1 3UJ, UK
[b] Department of Intestinal Imaging, St Mark's Hospital, Watford Road, Harrow, Middlesex HA1 3UJ, UK
[c] Department of Specialist Imaging, University College Hospital, 235 Euston Road, 2F Podium, London NW1 2BU, UK
* Corresponding author.
E-mail address: n.suzuki@imperial.ac.uk

Gastrointest Endoscopy Clin N Am 20 (2010) 565–572
doi:10.1016/j.giec.2010.03.011
1052-5157/10/$ – see front matter © 2010 Elsevier Inc. All rights reserved.

In day-to-day clinical practice, for CTC, any lesion that protrudes from the surrounding mucosa or results in focal thickening of the colonic wall, for example, an excavated lesion, is potentially visible (I, IIa, IIa+IIc) (**Figs. 1–4**). In contrast, truly flat lesions (IIb) or minimally depressed lesions (IIc) do not protrude and therefore are not generally detected by CTC. Fortunately, IIb and IIc lesions are rare, probably accounting for less than 3% of all neoplastic polyps.[13]

PERFORMANCE CHARACTERISTICS OF CTC

Over the last decade, numerous studies have compared performance of CTC and colonoscopy in the same patients, and the focus has been on detecting more common polypoid colorectal neoplasms. A recent meta-analysis[14] included 47 studies providing data on 10,546 patients. Per-polyp sensitivity of CTC for polyps smaller than 6 mm varied from 28% to 100%. The pooled, per-polyp sensitivities of CTC were 66% (95% confidence interval [CI], 64%–68%) overall for all polyps, 59% (95% CI, 56%–61%; range 16%–90%) for polyps 6 mm to 9 mm in size and 76% (95% CI, 73%–79%; range 50%–100%) for polyps larger than 9 mm. However, all analyses were statistically heterogenous, mainly because of different scanner technologies and protocols used in different studies. In single centers, CTC performance was equivalent to colonoscopy—one study[14,15] reported per-polyp sensitivity of 84% (lesions 6–9 mm) and 92% (≥10 mm) in 1233 asymptomatic adults. More recently, a large multicenter American College of Radiology Imaging Network (ACRIN study[16] of 2600 asymptomatic patients at 15 participating centers replicated similar large polyp sensitivity (84% for polyps 10 mm or larger). However, it has been noted for some time that detection of flat polyps may be very difficult at CTC,[5] and European Society of Gastrointestinal and Abdominal Radiology (ESGAR) CTC study group investigators found that most of the large polyps missed by expert observers were flat.[17]

Fidler and colleagues[6] were among the first to report detection of flat lesions by CTC in a high-risk population. Of 22 flat polyps detected at colonoscopy with mean size of 13 mm (4–35 mm), 14 were hyperplastic and 8, adenomas. Sensitivity for detection of all flat polyps (defined as height<half the long axis) by 3 reviewers was 15% to 65% and for flat adenomas, 13% to 100%. These results were encouraging, given the relatively inferior CTC technique used at that time (4-detector row scanner with 5-mm slice width, no automated insufflators or fecal tagging). In another series of 500 patients with 116 polyps, 16% were flat (defined as height<half the long axis); 3 of 9 (33%) flat lesions 5–9 mm in size could be detected prospectively, in contrast to 34 of 53 (64%) sessile and pedunculated polyps. Only 25% of flat lesions were detected even in retrospect.

Using the same definition and a specific technique (including fecal tagging and thinner slice width of 1.25–2.5 mm), Pickhardt and colleagues[18] showed that, prospectively, CTC detected 24 of 29 (82.8%) flat adenomas and 47 of 59 (80%) of all flat lesions 6 mm or larger. This was the first study to use 3-dimensional (3D) endoluminal fly-through for primary polyp detection and the authors thought this was a contributory factor to their relative success. In addition, 3D views are considered as the key metric when the ratio criterion (height ≤ half the long axis) is used in defining the flat lesions. Using the ratio criterion with 3D views enhanced reproducibility and decreased interobserver variability.[19]

However, minimally depressed lesions may be better detected with 2D images, because excavated lesions may grow more into the colonic wall than protrude into lumen harboring advanced histologic characteristics. These lesions may appear as a focal area of soft-tissue thickening in the wall.[20]

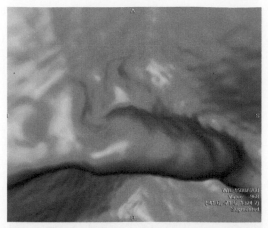

Fig. 1. Three-dimensional endoluminal image from virtual colonoscopy shows cecal lesion initially recognized as a thickened fold.

TECHNIQUE FOR DETECTING FLAT POLYPS AT CTC INCLUDING PITFALLS

Detection of flat neoplasia is hampered by a lack of direct mucosal visualization at CTC, such that subtle vascular and mucosal changes are not appreciated. There are 2 opportunities for radiologists to miss flat neoplasia: because of perceptual error (not seeing the polyp in the first place) or characterization (wrongly dismissing a flat polyp after initial detection).

Perceptual errors are exacerbated by suboptimal or poor quality technique, such that minimally elevated lesions are potentially hidden by bulbous folds, relatively thick mucosa in under-distended segments, or fecal/fluid residue. Intuitively, such error can be avoided by optimizing bowel preparation and colonic distension. Errors of characterization usually arise when the polyp candidate is subtle, when there is retained fecal residue or fluid, and if the polyp is only visible on one of the 2 scan acquisitions (because of segmental collapse or mucosa obscured by residue). One retrospective review[21] of 18 missed polyps containing 10 flat polyps showed that only 6 were

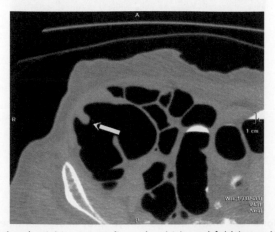

Fig. 2. Two-dimensional axial image confirms the thickened fold (*arrowhead*).

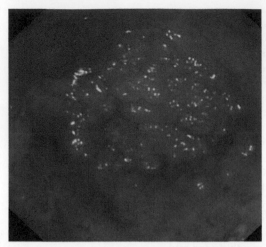

Fig. 3. Optical colonoscopy shows the cecal polyp, 0-IIa or LST-G (laterally spreading tumor-granular).

identified in retrospect and of these, 4 (67%) were considered to be missed because of poor bowel preparation.

Advice on protocols used to optimize flat polyp detection can be obtained from a recent international standards document, but locally, a combination of laxative and fecal-tagging agent or fecal tagging alone is used. Local audit at St Mark's has demonstrated that the shift to the use of fecal tagging has reduced examination failure rate from 4% to less than 1%. An anecdotal increase in flat polyp detection has been noted, although this may also be influenced by increasing experience of colonic distension and awareness of the need to detect flat neoplasia by their radiographers.

The following contribute to increasing reader confidence and accuracy when reporting flat neoplasms: (1) detection of the polyp on both scans (usually prone and supine) in a well-distended colorectum (usually facilitated by fecal tagging because dependent residue will therefore not obscure the polyp); (2) unchanged morphology between

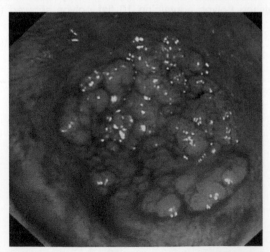

Fig. 4. Optical colonoscopy with the targeted dye spray (indigo carmine) highlighted the cecal flat lesion.

scans (usually best assessed on 3D displays); (3) use of abdominal CT window settings; (4) detection of transmural component, extraluminal hypervascularity, or lymphadenopathy when a flat polyp is malignant.

The role of intravenous contrast for detection of flat polyps is uncertain but its benefit is likely to be small and offset against the risk of the associated need to increase radiation dose. However, polyp enhancement may improve reader confidence, particularly where there is significant, untagged residue.[22,23]

In a small study of 10 patients with 18 flat lesions (9 adenomas, 3 advanced neoplastic lesions, and 6 hyperplasic polyps), Park and colleagues[24] reported the experience in detecting flat lesions on contrast enhanced 16-MDCT (multidetector CT) colonography with very narrow 1-mm slice. The authors detected less than half of the lesions and concluded that lesions must be 2 mm or greater in height and 7 mm or greater in diameter before they could be visualized.

COMPUTER-AIDED DETECTION OF FLAT NEOPLASMS

Computer-aided detection (CAD) is facilitating detection of colonic neoplasms and reducing interpretation times.[25–28] Conventional CAD systems have generally focused on detecting polypoid lesions (Paris 0-I lesions) using geometric morphologic and textural characteristics to distinguish polyps from normal structures in the colon, such as haustra folds, stool, air-liquid boundary, and ileocecal valve.

During the CAD processing steps, because of maximized sensitivity for polyps, a large number of candidate objects are generated by calculating 3D volumetric features within the CT image data or analysis of the surface of the colonic wall, for example, using shape and curvedness concentrations,[29] bloblike structures,[30] curvature surface normal overlap,[31] conformal colon flattening,[32] or polyp enhancing level sets.[33] Following this, various characteristics of the candidate polyps are calculated, and CAD eliminates as many false-positive (FP) candidates as possible while maintaining clinically acceptable levels of sensitivity.

The CAD detection process for flat neoplasm presents significant challenges. Flat neoplasms have smaller protrusions compared with polypoid lesions. Existing CAD systems may detect 0-IIa lesions but will not successfully detect 0-IIb (completely flat) or 0-IIc(depressed) lesions. Therefore, to achieve good detection capabilities, CAD methods must focus on subtle changes in intensity valid within the tissue structure of the colon wall rather than morphologic characteristics.

CTC WITH CAD IN FLAT NEOPLASMS: CLINICAL RESULTS

There has been limited CAD literature dealing specifically with detection of flat neoplasms. However, over the last few years, attention has switched to designing and testing algorithms for detecting such lesions.

Taylor and colleagues[34] presented the possibility that CAD detects flat early cancers when applied to 24 T1 colonic cancers endoscopically classified as flat. Retrospectively applying 3 settings of sphericity (0, 0.75, and 1), CAD (ColonCAD API 4.0, Medicsight plc, London, UK) detected 20 (83.3%),17 (70.8%), and 13 (54.1%) of the 24 cancers, respectively, with the mean total number of FP CAD marks per patient at each filter setting 36.5, 21.1, and 9.5, respectively. The lesions missed were predominantly classified as 0-IIa, with most of the 13 type IIa+IIc lesions detected. The study underlines the inevitable trade-off between maximizing lesion sensitivity and an acceptable FP rate.

Park examined a series of 23 flat lesions (height<2 mm) detected at colonoscopy.[35] Human readers detected 9 of 10 (90%) Tis or T1 flat adenocarcinomas (10–25 mm in size), but only 3 of 8 (37.5%) flat adenomas (size range 9–30 mm), and 0 of 5 (0%) flat non-neoplastic lesions. CAD (PEV version VC30A, Siemens Medical Solutions) detected these lesions at the rate of 90% (9 of 10), 12.5% (1 of 8), and 0% (0 of 5), respectively. Although the CAD did not enhance diagnostic yield for overall flat neoplastic lesions, the system showed high sensitivity in detection of flat colorectal cancers (CRCs) with cathartic bowel preparation and fecal tagging.

One prospective observer study using second-read CAD (Colon CAD, Phillips Medical Systems, Best, Netherlands) performed in 170 consecutive patients undergoing same-day colonoscopy was recently presented.[36] The CAD itself detected 72% of 58 polyps 6 to 9 mm in size and 60% of 30 polyps larger than 10 mm. Indeed, 13 of the 30 polyps larger than 10 mm were flat, of which 6 could not even be identified in retrospect by unblinded experienced readers. The addition of CAD improved per-polyp sensitivity for the flat lesions from 3 of 13 to 4 of 13. However, 60% of missed large flat lesions were not even visible in retrospect, demonstrating the major challenges faced by CAD and radiologist in detecting subtle flat neoplasms. It is clear that existing CAD system must be modified to facilitate detection of flat polyps.

Such modification has already been performed by some groups. Suzuki and colleagues[37] developed 3D massive-training artificial neural networks (MTANNs), which remove various types of FPs in CAD of polyps. It was designed to differentiate flat lesions from categories of FPs, namely rectal tubes, stools, folds, and ileocecal valve. They applied the new system to the CTC datasets obtained from 73 patients, of which 25 patients had 28 flat lesions (defined as height<3 mm or height<half the long axis). The MTANNs CAD detected 68% (19 of 28) of flat lesions, including 6 lesions previously missed by radiologists.[38] In addition, the new system improved the FP rate from an average of 3.1 (224/73) to 1.1(82/73) per patient without impairing original sensitivity.

A Korean group also developed a CAD referred to as the academic CAD system with improved per-polyp sensitivities in detection of flat lesions compared with 2 commercially available CAD systems, namely Computer Assisted Reader (CAR) (version 3.02, Philips Healthcare) and Polyp Enhanced View (PEV) (version B10A, Siemens Healthcare).[39] Per-polyp sensitivities as determined with the CAR, PEV, and the academic CAD system for flat lesions were 51.5%, 57.6%, and 81.8%, respectively, whereas the number of FPs was not significantly different (average number of FPs 3.8, 2.6, and 4.6 in CAR, PEV, and their academic CAD system, respectively).

SUMMARY

As a proportion of CRC develops from flat neoplasms, a consistently higher sensitivity of CTC for flat neoplasms needs to be achieved. Optimal bowel preparation and distension, fecal tagging, and experienced interpretation using a combination of 3D and 2D views should lead to higher CTC sensitivity for conspicuous flat elevated and depressed lesions. There is evidence that some existing computer-aided diagnosis (CAD) systems have reasonable detection characteristics despite being focused on more common polypoid neoplasms. Modification of CAD for flat neoplasms will, without doubt, further enhance performance of CTC and establish it as a viable alternative to colonoscopy for CRC screening.

REFERENCES

1. Fenlon HM, Nunes DP, Schroy PC III, et al. A comparison of virtual and conventional colonoscopy for the detection of colorectal polyps. N Engl J Med 1999; 341(20):1496–503.

2. Pineau BC, Paskett ED, Chen GJ, et al. Virtual colonoscopy using oral contrast compared with colonoscopy for the detection of patients with colorectal polyps. Gastroenterology 2003;125(2):304–10.
3. Yee J, Akerkar GA, Hung RK, et al. Colorectal neoplasia: performance characteristics of CT colonography for detection in 300 patients. Radiology 2001;219(3):685–92.
4. Pickhardt PJ, Nugent PA, Choi JR, et al. Flat colorectal lesions in asymptomatic adults: implications for screening with CT virtual colonoscopy. AJR Am J Roentgenol 2004;183(5):1343–7.
5. Macari M, Bini EJ, Jacobs SL, et al. Filling defects at CT colonography: pseudo- and diminutive lesions (the good), polyps (the bad), flat lesions, masses, and carcinomas (the ugly). Radiographics 2003;23(5):1073–91.
6. Fidler JL, Johnson CD, MacCarty RL, et al. Detection of flat lesions in the colon with CT colonography. Abdom Imaging 2002;27(3):292–300.
7. Soetikno RM, Kaltenbach T, Rouse RV, et al. Prevalence of nonpolypoid (flat and depressed) colorectal neoplasms in asymptomatic and symptomatic adults. JAMA 2008;299(9):1027–35.
8. Burling D, Halligan S, Altman DG, et al. Polyp measurement and size categorisation by CT colonography: effect of observer experience in a multi-centre setting. Eur Radiol 2006;16(8):1737–44.
9. Kim DH, Pickhardt PJ, Taylor AJ, et al. CT colonography versus colonoscopy for the detection of advanced neoplasia. N Engl J Med 2007;357(14):1403–12.
10. Paris Workshop participants. The Paris endoscopic classification of superficial neoplastic lesions: esophagus, stomach, and colon. Gastrointest Endosc 2003; 58:S3–43
11. Sawada T, Hojo K, Moriya Y. Colonoscopic management of focal and early colorectal carcinoma. Baillieres Clin Gastroenterol 1989;3(3):627–45.
12. Zalis ME, Barish MA, Choi JR, et al. CT colonography reporting and data system: a consensus proposal. Radiology 2005;236(1):3–9.
13. Suzuki N, Price AB, Talbot IC, et al. Flat colorectal neoplasms and the impact of the revised Vienna classification on their reporting: a case-control study in UK and Japanese patients. Scand J Gastroenterol 2006;41(7):812–9.
14. Chaparro M, Gisbert JP, Del Campo L, et al. Accuracy of computed tomographic colonography for the detection of polyps and colorectal tumors: a systematic review and meta-analysis. Digestion 2009;80(1):1–17.
15. Pickhardt PJ, Choi JR, Hwang I, et al. Computed tomographic virtual colonoscopy to screen for colorectal neoplasia in asymptomatic adults. N Engl J Med 2003;349(23):2191–200.
16. Johnson CD, Chen MH, Toledano AY, et al. Accuracy of CT colonography for detection of large adenomas and cancers. N Engl J Med 2008;359(12):1207–17.
17. European Society of Gastrointestinal and Abdominal Radiology CT Colonography Group Investigators. Effect of directed training on reader performance for CT colonography: multicenter study. Radiology 2007;242(1):152–61.
18. Pickhardt PJ, Choi JH. Electronic cleansing and stool tagging in CT colonography: advantages and pitfalls with primary three-dimensional evaluation. AJR Am J Roentgenol 2003;181(3):799–805.
19. Lostumbo A, Wanamaker C, Tsai J, et al. Comparison of 2D and 3D views for evaluation of flat lesions in CT colonography. Acad Radiol 2010;17(1):39–47.
20. Fidler J, Johnson C. Flat polyps of the colon: accuracy of detection by CT colonography and histologic significance. Abdom Imaging 2009;34(2):157–71.
21. MacCarty RL, Johnson CD, Fletcher JG, et al. Occult colorectal polyps on CT colonography: implications for surveillance. AJR Am J Roentgenol 2006;186(5):1380–3.

22. Morrin MM, Raptopoulos V. Contrast-enhanced CT colonography. Semin Ultrasound CT MR 2001;22(5):420–4.
23. Park SH, Ha HK, Kim MJ, et al. False-negative results at multi-detector row CT colonography: multivariate analysis of causes for missed lesions. Radiology 2005;235(2):495–502.
24. Park SH, Ha HK, Kim AY, et al. Flat polyps of the colon: detection with 16-MDCT colonography–preliminary results. AJR Am J Roentgenol 2006;186(6):1611–7.
25. Mang T, Peloschek P, Plank C, et al. Effect of computer-aided detection as a second reader in multidetector-row CT colonography. Eur Radiol 2007;17(10):2598–607.
26. Nappi J, Dachman AH, MacEneaney P, et al. Automated knowledge-guided segmentation of colonic walls for computerized detection of polyps in CT colonography. J Comput Assist Tomogr 2002;26(4):493–504.
27. Summers RM, Yao J, Pickhardt PJ, et al. Computed tomographic virtual colonoscopy computer-aided polyp detection in a screening population. Gastroenterology 2005;129(6):1832–44.
28. Halligan S, Altman DG, Mallett S, et al. Computed tomographic colonography: assessment of radiologist performance with and without computer-aided detection. Gastroenterology 2006;131(6):1690–9.
29. Yoshida H, Masutani Y, MacEneaney P, et al. Computerized detection of colonic polyps at CT colonography on the basis of volumetric features: pilot study. Radiology 2002;222(2):327–36.
30. Kim SH, Lee JM, Lee JG, et al. Computer-aided detection of colonic polyps at CT colonography using a Hessian matrix-based algorithm: preliminary study. AJR Am J Roentgenol 2007;189(1):41–51.
31. Kiss G, Van Cleynenbreugel J, Thomeer M, et al. Computer-aided diagnosis in virtual colonography via combination of surface normal and sphere fitting methods. Eur Radiol 2002;12(1):77–81.
32. Hong W, Qiu F, Kaufman A. A pipeline for computer aided polyp detection. IEEE Trans Vis Comput Graph 2006;12(5):861–8.
33. Konukoglu E, Acar B, Paik DS, et al. Polyp enhancing level set evolution of colon wall: method and pilot study. IEEE Trans Med Imaging 2007;26(12):1649–56.
34. Taylor SA, Iinuma G, Saito Y, et al. CT colonography: computer-aided detection of morphologically flat T1 colonic carcinoma. Eur Radiol 2008;18(8):1666–73.
35. Park SH, Kim SY, Lee SS, et al. Sensitivity of CT colonography for nonpolypoid colorectal lesions interpreted by human readers and with computer-aided detection. AJR Am J Roentgenol 2009;193(1):70–8.
36. de Vries AH, Jensch S, Liedenbaum MH, et al. Does a computer-aided detection algorithm in a second read paradigm enhance the performance of experienced computed tomography colonography readers in a population of increased risk? Eur Radiol 2009;19(4):941–50.
37. Suzuki K, Yoshida H, Nappi J, et al. Mixture of expert 3D massive-training ANNs for reduction of multiple types of false positives in CAD for detection of polyps in CT colonography. Med Phys 2008;35(2):694–703.
38. Doshi T, Rusinak D, Halvorsen RA, et al. CT colonography: false-negative interpretations. Radiology 2007;244(1):165–73.
39. Lee MW, Kim SH, Park HS, et al. An anthropomorphic phantom study of computer-aided detection performance for polyp detection on CT colonography: a comparison of commercially and academically available systems. AJR Am J Roentgenol 2009;193(2):445–54.

Genetic Aspects of Non-Polypoid Colorectal Neoplasms

Lyn Sue Kahng, MD

KEYWORDS

- Colorectal cancer • Non-polypoid colorectal neoplasms
- Research • Molecular genetics

Rapid advances in colorectal cancer (CRC) research continue to provide a deeper understanding of the genetic underpinnings of tumor behavior and the ways in which genotype and phenotype may correlate with neoplastic morphology and clinical prognosis. Genetic alterations in the development of colorectal cancer (CRC) are now known to involve different pathways. They initially were characterized in the adenoma–carcinoma sequence, where, in a model first proposed by Fearon and Vogelstein,[1] CRC develops as mutations accumulate in a stepwise manner. Characteristic genetic changes include the progressive loss of wild-type tumor suppressor genes; frequently loss of heterozygosity (LOH) at chromosome 5q (APC), 17p (p53), and 18q (DCC/SMAD locus); and activating point mutations of K-ras. Other cancers arise through mutations in the DNA mismatch repair system, as seen in Lynch syndrome, and display microsatellite instability. In addition to these genetic changes, epigenetic modifications have emerged as a crucial factor in CRC development, specifically aberrant promoter hypermethylation, which affects key tumor suppressor genes (CpG island methylator phenotype, or CIMP). The type and degree of genetic instability as well as CIMP status in CRCs allows their classification into different molecular subtypes.[2]

It is of great interest how pathways of tumor development differ; for example, the genetics of the serrated adenoma pathway are being elucidated and are described separately in this issue. The lower abundance of flat neoplasms has provided more limited and sometimes conflicting data in understanding the genetic factors that give rise to them. Still, genetic differences between non-polypoid and polypoid neoplasms were already proposed as early as 1994 and continue to be explored in the context of newly discovered mechanisms of tumorigenesis for various lesions including flat adenomas, carcinomas, de novo carcinoma, and laterally spreading tumors.

Section of Digestive Diseases and Nutrition, University of Illinois at Chicago and Jesse Brown VA Medical Center, Chicago, IL 60612, USA
E-mail address: lynsue@uic.edu

Gastrointest Endoscopy Clin N Am 20 (2010) 573–578
doi:10.1016/j.giec.2010.03.004
1052-5157/10/$ – see front matter. Published by Elsevier Inc.

K-*ras* MUTATIONS AND THE RAS PATHWAY

The mutations best-characterized in non-polypoid lesions are those in K-*ras*. Several studies, including the following, have suggested that K-*ras* mutations are rarer in non-polypoid lesions than polypoid ones. For example, Yamagata and colleagues found that K-*ras* mutations could be found in only 23% of flat adenomas, versus 67% of polypoid adenomas. Kaneko and colleagues[3] similarly studied a series of 42 carcinomas. They found that p53 overexpression did not differ between the two morphologies but that the non-polypoid cancers lacked K-*ras* mutations, whereas they were present in 44% of the polypoid cancers. Olschwang and colleagues[4] analyzed a series of 44 flat colorectal neoplasms for microsatellite instability and mutations in *APC*, K-*ras*, and *TGF-RII* and found that only K-*ras* mutations had a lower frequency than in polypoid neoplasms. Umetani and colleagues[5] found K-*ras* mutations in none of their superficial depressed adenomas but 31% of polypoid adenomas.

Laterally spreading tumors (LSTs) also have been analyzed, although the results are less clear. For K-*ras* mutations, Hiraoka and colleagues[6] and Mukawa and colleagues[7] found a lower prevalence in flat nongranular lesions (16% and 26% respectively) versus granular lesions that are more protruded (78% and 77% respectively). In contrast, Takahashi and colleagues[8] found that although K-*ras* mutation was present in 35% of flat-type LSTs, it was only present in 13% of protruded-type adenomas.

In addition to concluding that K-*ras* mutations correlate with polypoid growth, Yashiro and colleagues[9] also found an association of LOH at chromosome 3p with cancers of the de novo type, a region known to contain multiple tumor suppressors or related genes, including *MLH1*, *β-catenin*, *TGFBR2*, and *RASSF1A*. *RASSF1A* is a member of a relatively recently discovered family of proteins with tumor suppressor functions, for which epigenetic inactivation by promoter hypermethylation has been described in a wide variety of cancers.[10,11] Although almost universal in some cancers such as breast or small cell lung cancer, *RASSF1A* methylation is less frequent in CRC.[10] Van Engeland and colleagues[12] found that 45 of 222 (20%) sporadic CRCs had *RASSF1A* methylation, and of six normal epithelial samples from cancer patients, only one had *RASSF1A* methylation. Oliveira and colleagues[13] found a higher frequency (22 of 51 cases, or 43%), studying polypoid tumors with microsatellite instability. Sakamoto and colleagues[14] investigated the frequency in 48 flat tumors comprising 39 early carcinomas and nine high-grade dysplasias; 39 of 48 (81.3%) had *RASSF1A* methylation, but only 7 of 48 (14.6%) had K-*ras* mutations. In the 39 cases of tumors with *RASSF1A* methylation, 19 (49%) also showed *RASSF1A* methylation in morphologically normal mucosa. It is unclear whether this represents an abnormal background giving rise to tumors, versus a field effect. More data are needed to clarify the roles of these family members, as a separate study by Noda and colleagues[15] showed a low (16.4%) incidence of *RASSF1A* methylation in all tumors, with no difference between flat and polypoid lesions. Analysis of *RASSF2* methylation has been found in 43% of tumors in another series, again with no difference between flat and protruded neoplasms.[16] Still, alternate pathways to perturbing RAS signaling may be present in flat colonic neoplasms and their background mucosa.

ROLE OF APC AND LOH AT CHROMOSOME 17P

There are differing data regarding APC, as Umetani and colleagues[5] found that in addition to a lower K-*ras* frequency, APC mutation was also less frequent in flat versus polypoid adenomas (13% vs 43%, encompassing both depressed and elevated flat adenomas vs polypoid ones) although the frequency was similar in carcinomas.

On the other hand, Kaneko and colleagues[3] found that although the rate of APC mutation in polypoid versus non-polypoid carcinomas was similar, the types of mutations differed. Non-polypoid carcinomas completely lacked frameshift mutations that were found in 66% of polypoid carcinomas, thus leading the authors to propose that different types of APC mutations could influence tumor morphology and development.

In a similar vein, several groups have analyzed loss of heterozygosity at multiple loci, most notably chromosome 17p. Several studies have concluded that LOH at chromosome 17p or p53 overexpression occurs with similar frequency in both flat and polypoid neoplasms.[9,17–20] LOH at 17p, however, has been found to be the most frequent (92%) of multiple LOH found in a series of flat tumors,[21] and Mueller and colleagues[22] found LOH at 17p in 73% of de novo cancers versus 37% of ex-adenoma cancers.

OTHER MOLECULAR CORRELATES OF TUMOR BEHAVIOR

With respect to other markers, Wlodarczyk and colleagues[23] also found more de novo cancers with decreased E-cadherin expression and extensive stromelysin-3 expression. It has recently been proposed that CD10, β-catenin, and mucin expression may correlate with flat tumor morphology and prognosis also.[24] CD10 is a marker that in CRC correlates with a higher incidence of venous invasion or liver metastasis, although a causal relationship has not been established. In contrast, the absence of MUC5AC may be important. MUC5AC is not normally expressed in the colon, but frequently is expressed de novo in adenomas and colorectal cancers. It has been suggested that MUC5AC negativity correlates with higher metastatic potential and poorer prognosis, and it may be differentially expressed in MSI-H (77%) versus MSS cancers (28%).[25] Finally, the β-catenin signaling pathway has key roles in development and cancer, where the protein is often stabilized due to APC or β-catenin mutation and aberrant signaling ensues. Koga and colleagues[24] performed immunohistochemistry to assess CD10, nuclear β-catenin, MUC2, and MUC5AC in 111 flat colorectal neoplasms and 96 polypoid ones. CD10 was found in 50% of flat low-grade neoplasia (LGN) but 0% of polypoid LGN, as well as 59% of flat high-grade neoplasia versus 33% of polypoid neoplasia. Invasive lesions had, respectively, 51% and 39% CD10 positivity. Nuclear β-catenin was found in 86% of non-polypoid LGN versus 58% of polypoid LGN, but similar percentages of HGN and invasive neoplasia. For non-polypoid versus polypoid lesions, MUC5AC was present in 25% versus 50% of LGNs; 0% versus 28% of HGN; and 3% versus 32% of invasive neoplasia. Markers of more aggressive phenotype therefore may be present at an earlier stage in flat neoplasms compared with polypoid ones.

MICROSATELLITE INSTABILITY AND METHYLATION

Microsatellite instability has been observed by Kaneko and colleagues[3] to be similar between polypoid and non-polypoid carcinomas (16% of tumors of each type). In a different study, however, Ogawa and colleagues[26] found non-polypoid cancers to have a higher level of MSI with chromosome 17 markers (33%) than polypoid cancers (10%); in the stroma, these numbers were 8% and 4% respectively. Of 16 flat/depressed lesions described by Kinney and colleagues[27] in an American series, five (31%) displayed MSI, similar to the Ogawa study. Thus MSI is not a predominant hallmark of these flat lesions, although further comparisons between non-polypoid and polypoid lesions will show whether there are reproducible differences between the two. Methylation may be important in their development, as Hiraoka and colleagues[6] found CIMP-high status less likely in flat LST (8%) than granular LST (61%), and Taka-hashi and colleagues[8] observed a trend toward less gene methylation in flat-type adenomas than protruded-type.

FUTURE DIRECTIONS: GENOME-WIDE TRANSCRIPTIONAL ANALYSIS AND DEVELOPMENT OF ANIMAL MODELS

Can animal models and gene expression analyses shed additional light on the development of flat neoplasms? A microarray analysis has been performed on 12 patients with flat adenomas, using adjacent normal mucosa as a control.[28] The authors found that 180 genes were differentially expressed, and the expression profiles of right colon lesions were different from those in the left colon. Three genes, *MMP7*, *CDH3*, and *DUOX2*, were up-regulated more than 10-fold in flat adenomas. The authors correlated this transcriptional upregulation with increased immunohistochemical staining of MMP7 and CDH3 in lesions. Real-time polymerase chain reaction analyzing expression of these three genes in polypoid adenomas showed that their levels of expression were elevated over those in normal mucosa, but were still 27% to 58% lower than in flat adenomas. The roles in development of neoplasia are still not fully understood, but it has been suggested that MMP7 overexpression correlates with more advanced adenoma histology, and elevated serum levels with poor prognosis in CRC.[29,30] This study is interesting in identifying candidates for further study as well as adding to the literature suggesting differential gene expression in the proximal and distal colon for both normal and neoplastic mucosa.[31]

One group has reported that in the azoxymethane mouse model of CRC, genetic background can lead to different polyp morphologies; 19% of tumors in KK/HIJ mice are flat, whereas 83% are flat in I/LNJ mice.[32] The authors performed serial colonoscopy and histologic analysis, finding that flat polyps continued to grow without becoming more exophytic, and protuberant polyps were overtly raised from first observation. One difference between this study and work described previously was that all azoxymethane-induced flat cancers had adenomatous components, and were thus not de novo cancers. In addition, both flat and polypoid lesions had a similarly low frequency of K-*ras* mutation (7%), lower than normally found in human polypoid neoplasms. Despite these contrasts, it is an interesting model in which to study the influence of genetics on carcinogenesis and morphology.

SUMMARY

Colorectal cancer is now understood to be a heterogeneous disease arising through multiple possible pathways. Elucidating the genetic factors controlling molecular phenotype, morphology, histology, and prognosis of different tumor types continues to be a challenge.

Non-polypoid colonic neoplasms provide exciting opportunities for ongoing study of their underlying genetic abnormalities and molecular phenotypes. The varied data from different groups, however, highlight the need for further studies in different populations. With growing awareness of non-polypoid lesions in Western populations, larger series will no doubt be forthcoming to facilitate this research.

REFERENCES

1. Fearon ER, Vogelstein B. A genetic model for colorectal tumorigenesis. Cell 1990; 61:759–67.

2. Jass JR. Classification of colorectal cancer based on correlation of clinical, morphological, and molecular features. Histopathology 2007;50:113–30.
3. Kaneko K, Fujii T, Kato S, et al. Growth patterns and genetic changes of colorectal carcinoma. Jpn J Clin Oncol 1998;28:196–201.
4. Olschwang S, Slezak P, Roze M, et al. Somatically acquired genetic alterations in flat colorectal neoplasias. Int J Cancer 1998;77:366–9.
5. Umetani N, Sasaki S, Masaki T, et al. Involvement of APC and K-*ras* mutation in nonpolypoid colorectal tumorigenesis. Br J Cancer 2000;82:9–15.
6. Hiraoka S, Kato J, Tatsukawa M, et al. Laterally spreading type of colorectal adenoma exhibits a unique methylation phenotype and K-*ras* mutations. Gastroenterology 2006;131:379–89.
7. Mukawa K, Fujii S, Takeda J, et al. Analysis of K-*ras* mutations and expression of cyclooxygenase-2 and gastrin protein in laterally spreading tumors. J Gastroenterol Hepatol 2005;20:1584–90.
8. Takahashi T, Nosho K, Yamamoto H, et al. Flat-type colorectal advanced adenomas (laterally spreading tumors) have different genetic and epigenetic alterations from protruded-type advanced adenomas. Mod Pathol 2007;20:139–47.
9. Yashiro M, Carethers JM, Laghi L, et al. Genetic pathways in the evolution of morphologically distinct colorectal neoplasms. Cancer Res 2001;61:2676–83.
10. Donninger H, Vos MD, Clark GJ. The *RASSF1A* tumor suppressor. J Cell Sci 2007;120:3163–72.
11. Richter AM, Pfeifer GP, Dammann RH. The RASSF proteins in cancer; from epigenetic silencing to functional characterization. Biochim Biophys Acta 2009;1796:114–28.
12. van Engeland M, Roemen GM, Brink M, et al. K-*ras* mutations and *RASSF1A* promoter methylation in colorectal cancer. Oncogene 2002;21:3792–5.
13. Oliveira C, Velho S, Domingo E, et al. Concomitant *RASSF1A* hypermethylation and *KRAS/BRAF* mutations occur preferentially in MSI sporadic colorectal cancer. Oncogene 2005;24:7630–4.
14. Sakamoto N, Terai T, Ajioka Y, et al. Frequent hypermethylation of RASSF1A in early flat-type colorectal tumors. Oncogene 2004;23:8900–7.
15. Noda H, Kato Y, Yoshikawa H, et al. Frequent involvement of ras-signaling pathways in both polypoid-type and flat-type early stage colorectal cancers. J Exp Clin Cancer Res 2006;25:235–42.
16. Nosho K, Yamamoto H, Takahashi T, et al. Genetic and epigenetic profiling in early colorectal tumors and prediction of invasive potential in pT1 (early invasive) colorectal cancers. Carcinogenesis 2007;28:1364–70.
17. Hirata I, Wang FY, Murano M, et al. Histopathological and genetic differences between polypoid and nonpolypoid submucosal colorectal carcinoma. World J Gastroenterol 2007;13:2048–52.
18. Rubio CA, Rodensjo M. Mutation of p53 tumor suppressor gene in flat neoplastic lesions of the colorectal mucosa. Dis Colon Rectum 1996;39:143–7.
19. Saitoh Y, Waxman I, West AB, et al. Prevalence and distinctive biologic features of flat colorectal adenomas in a North American population. Gastroenterology 2001;120:1657–65.
20. Watanabe T, Muto T. Colorectal carcinogenesis based on molecular biology of early colorectal cancer, with special reference to nonpolypoid (superficial) lesions. World J Surg 2000;24:1091–7.
21. Orita H, Sakamoto N, Ajioka Y, et al. Allelic loss analysis of early stage flat-type colorectal tumors. Ann Oncol 2006;17:43–9.

22. Mueller JD, Haegle N, Keller G, et al. Loss of heterozygosity and microsatellite instability in de novo versus ex-adenoma carcinomas of the colorectum. Am J Pathol 1998;153:1977–84.
23. Wlodarczyk J, Bethke B, Mueller E, et al. A comparative study of E-cadherin and stromelysin-3 expression in de novo and ex adenoma carcinoma of the colorectum. Virchows Arch 2001;439:756–61.
24. Koga Y, Yao T, Hirahashi M, et al. Flat adenoma–carcinoma sequence with high-malignancy potential as demonstrated by CD10 and beta-catenin expression: a different pathway from the polypoid adenoma–carcinoma sequence. Histopathology 2008;52:569–77.
25. Byrd JC, Bresalier RS. Mucins and mucin binding proteins in colorectal cancer. Cancer Metastasis Rev 2004;23:77–99.
26. Ogawa T, Yoshida T, Tsuruta T, et al. Genetic instability on chromosome 17 in the epithelium of non-polypoid colorectal carcinomas compared to polypoid lesions. Cancer Sci 2006;97:1335–42.
27. Kinney TP, Merel N, Hart J, et al. Microsatellite analysis of sporadic flat and depressed lesions of the colon. Dig Dis Sci 2005;50:327–30.
28. Kita H, Hikichi Y, Hikami K, et al. Differential gene expression between flat adenoma and normal mucosa in the colon in a microarray analysis. J Gastroenterol 2006;41:1053–63.
29. Kirimlioglu H, Kirimlioglu V, Yilmaz S, et al. Role of matrix metalloproteinase-7 in colorectal adenomas. Dig Dis Sci 2006;51:2068–72.
30. Maurel J, Nadal C, Garcia-Albeniz X, et al. Serum matrix metalloproteinase 7 levels identifies poor prognosis advanced colorectal cancer patients. Int J Cancer 2007;121:1066–71.
31. Birkenkamp-Demtroder K, Olesen SH, Sorensen FB, et al. Differential gene expression in colon cancer of the caecum versus the sigmoid and rectosigmoid. Gut 2005;54:374–84.
32. Uronis JM, Herfarth HH, Rubinas TC, et al. Flat colorectal cancers are genetically determined and progress to invasion without going through a polypoid stage. Cancer Res 2007;67:11594–600.

Targeted Imaging of Flat and Depressed Colonic Neoplasms

Thomas D. Wang, MD, PhD[a,b,*]

KEYWORDS

- Molecular imaging • Colonic neoplasms
- Dysplasia • Flat and depressed • Targets

The presence of non-polypoid colorectal neoplasms is drawing significantly greater attention in the effort to improve methods for the early detection of colorectal cancer.[1] These lesions are much more difficult to identify on conventional white light endoscopy because their architectural changes are subtle and can be difficult to distinguish from that of normal colonic mucosa. By comparison, non-polypoid lesions can appear slightly elevated, completely flat, or slightly depressed.[2] In particular, depressed lesions are the most difficult to detect, and have the highest malignant potential. Recent studies have reported a significant miss rate on colonoscopy, and subsequent endoscopic therapy requires an accurate definition of tumor margins. Molecular imaging is a novel, emerging methodology that identifies functional properties of tissue based on the specific molecular signature of the mucosa. This field has been driven in part by recent advances in our understanding of tumor genetics that allow for future personalized oncological therapy. New molecular probes and imaging instruments are being developed to visualize the unique patterns of molecular expression in the mucosa of the digestive tract. Progress is being made in a number of imaging platforms that target biomolecules that are over expressed in cancer. Moreover, novel imaging instruments, including fluorescence endoscopy and confocal microscopy, are being developed to provide wide-area surveillance and microscopic examination, respectively.

This work was supported by Grant Nos. U54 CA136429 and P50 CA93990 from the National Institutes of Health.

The author has nothing to disclose.

[a] Division of Gastroenterology and Hepatology, Department of Medicine, University of Michigan School of Medicine, 109 Zina Pitcher Place, BSRB 1522, Ann Arbor, MI 48109, USA

[b] Department of Biomedical Engineering, University of Michigan, 109 Zina Pitcher Place, BSRB 1522, Ann Arbor, MI 48109, USA

* Division of Gastroenterology and Hepatology, Department of Medicine, University of Michigan School of Medicine, 109 Zina Pitcher Place, BSRB 1522, Ann Arbor, MI 48109.

E-mail address: thomaswa@umich.edu

MOLECULAR PROBES

Molecular probes are used to reveal subtle molecular changes in the cells and tissues that are present even in the absence of structural abnormalities, and can identify the over expression of targets to guide therapy in addition to performing diagnostics. Even with the highest resolution optical imaging instruments, exogenous probes are needed to observe important biologic processes, including up-regulation of growth factors, presence of proteolytic enzymes, and expression of cell adhesion molecules, that drive the progression of disease.[3] These probes are fluorescent-labeled for enhancing image contrast on endoscopic detection and for overcoming background tissue auto-fluorescence. Specific applications include performing in vivo lesion characterization, providing risk stratification, and assessing response to specific therapies. Further-more, because disease develops from genetic changes that are unique to each individual patient, targeting of specific molecular mechanisms can be used to tailor therapy that will maximize efficacy.

The antibody is one of the first targeting agents used for optical imaging, and is best suited for detection of extracellular targets and cell-surface receptors. These Y-shaped gamma globulins (IgG) express light chains on the distal end of either arm that binds selectively to over expressed targets with high affinity and specificity. The light chains can accommodate a large number of different amino acid sequences, resulting in a high diversity. Antibodies have been developed for several molecular targets that have great therapeutic relevance, including human epidermal growth factor receptor (ERBB2) and epidermal growth factor receptor (EGFR). However, there are several disadvantages for use of whole antibodies in molecular imaging. Their long circulatory half-life results in greater nonspecific binding, and increased tumor vascular permeability often produces a high background level. Moreover, they may elicit an immune reaction with repeated use, and are costly to produce in large quantities.

Peptides have tremendous advantages for performing targeted detection and therapy in the colon because of their high diversity, rapid binding kinetics, and potential for deep penetration into diseased mucosa. In addition, peptides can be labeled easily, are generally nontoxic, and are not immunogenic. These molecular probes have been developed using techniques of phage display, a powerful combinatorial method that uses recombinant DNA technology to generate a library of peptides that bind preferentially to cell surface targets. The protein coat of bacteriophage, such as the filamentous M13 or T7, is genetically engineered to express a very large number ($>10^9$) of different peptides with unique sequences. Selection of sequences with high-affinity binding is then performed by biopanning the library against cultured cells that over express desired targets. The DNA sequences are then recovered and used to synthesize the candidate peptides. Techniques of phage display have been successfully used to identify peptides that bind preferentially to dysplastic colonic mucosa and not to normal mucosa by employing a biopanning strategy that uses cultured cells and freshly excised normal and dysplastic tissues.

IMAGING INSTRUMENTS

Novel endoscopic instruments that are sensitive to fluorescence are needed to perform wide-area surveillance as well as microscopic examination. The endoscope, shown in **Fig. 1**, has 2 detectors for collecting white light (WL) images and fluores-cence separately.[4] The white light image is collected by the center detector, and the fluorescence image is collected by a second detector located near the periphery. Illumination for both modes is delivered through the 2 fiber light guides. In the WL

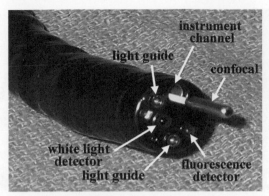

Fig. 1. Novel imaging instruments. Wide-area endoscopic images are collected by fluorescence detector, and microscopic images are acquired by confocal miniprobe. These instruments can be used together to guide "optical biopsy."

mode, the full visible spectrum (400 to 700 nm) is provided, whereas in the fluorescence mode, a second filter wheel enters the illumination path, and provides fluorescence excitation in the 395- to 475-nm spectral band. In addition, illumination from 525 to 575 nm provides reflected light in the green spectral regime centered at 550 nm. The fluorescence image is collected by the peripherally located charge-coupled device (CCD) detector that has a 490- to 625-nm band pass filter for blocking the excitation light. Because the increased vasculature in neoplastic mucosa absorbs autofluorescence, it appears with decreased intensity.

The confocal miniprobe (Cellvizio-GI, Paris, France), shown in **Fig. 1**, consists of a flexible fiber-imaging bundle that uses a 488-nm laser for excitation light.[5] The beam is scanned by a set of rotating mirrors located in the instrument unit. A microlens located at the distal end of the miniprobe focuses the beam into the tissue as well as collects the returning fluorescence. Fluorescence is collected by the same fibers and is transmitted back to the detector. The cores of the fiber act as collection pinholes for rejecting out-of-focus light to perform optical sectioning. A long-pass filter rejects the excitation light, and fluorescence is detected with an avalanche photodiode. The small outer diameter (<3 mm) allows for easy passage of the miniprobe through the instrument channel of the endoscope, allowing for the wide-area view to accurately guide placement onto the mucosal surface. Separate miniprobes provide distinct working distances up to 100 μm, and have a resolution between 1.0 and 3.5 μm. Images are collected in a horizontal plane (en face) at 12 frames per second with a field of view of approximately 600 μm. The frame rate is adequate to achieve consistent images with little interference from motion artifacts.

IMAGING RESULTS

Clinical imaging has been performed with fluorescence-labeled peptides to evaluate the spatial extent of non-polypoid lesions in the colon. In **Fig. 2A**, a standard white light endoscopic image shows a sessile mass approximately 10 mm in size found to be carcinoma-in-situ (CIS) on histology. The fluorescence image, shown in **Fig. 2B**, collected after topical administration of the fluorescent-labeled peptide "VRPMPLQ" reveals increased intensity at the site of the lesion compared with that of the adjacent normal mucosa.[6] Moreover, the presence of neoplastic crypts can be validated on the cellular level with confocal microscopy. A standard white light image of a dysplastic

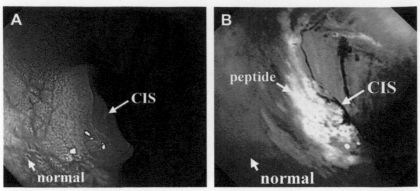

Fig. 2. Targeted endoscopic imaging. (*A*) A 10-mm lesion (carcinoma-in-situ) is seen on white light endoscopy. (*B*) Targeted image using topical administration of fluorescent-labeled peptides reveals tumor margins.

polyp is shown in **Fig. 3**A. The confocal image in **Fig. 3**B, collected after topical administration of the fluorescent-labeled peptide VRPMPLQ, reveals increased fluorescence intensity from the colonocytes in dysplastic but not in the normal crypts.[7] These images demonstrate the importance of targeted imaging and its future role in the management of non-polypoid colonic neoplasms. Because of their morphology and indistinct margins, these lesions are difficult to remove in entirety under white light guidance alone. The addition of the peptide-stained images provides functional information about neoplastic target over expression that can help improve the completeness of resection.

FUTURE CHALLENGES

There exists an important clinical need for more accurate endoscopic detection of flat and depressed colonic neoplasms to improve our effectiveness in performing cancer screening and surveillance. These lesions often contain severe dysplasia and are

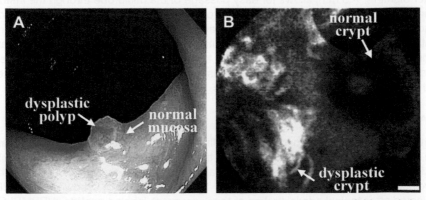

Fig. 3. Targeted confocal imaging. (*A*) A dysplastic polyp sits on a colonic fold consisting of normal mucosa. (*B*) Confocal image following administration of fluorescent-labeled peptides demonstrates preferential binding to dysplastic crypt (*left*) in comparison with adjacent normal crypt (*right*) (scale bar 20 μm).

aggressive in nature. In addition, high specificity is needed to distinguish neoplastic from non-neoplastic lesions that may include normal mucosa, hyperplasic polyps, colitis foci, and scar tissue. These lesions can be small (<10 mm in dimension) and patchy, thus techniques of wide-area surveillance and high magnification are needed. Molecular imaging represents an exciting new methodology that targets over expressed biomolecules in cancer that can identify and outline flat and depressed lesions on routine colonoscopy. A variety of probe platforms and imaging instruments are being developed to use fluorescence to enhance image contrast. Future advancements include the detection of important cell surface targets, such as EGFR and c-MET, to perform image-guided therapy in addition to diagnosis.

REFERENCES

1. Jaramillo E, Watanabe M, Slezak P, et al. Flat neoplastic lesions of the colon and rectum detected by high-resolution video endoscopy and chromoscopy. Gastrointest Endosc 1995;42:114–22.
2. Soetikno RM, Kaltenbach T, Rouse RV, et al. Prevalence of nonpolypoid (flat and depressed) colorectal neoplasms in asymptomatic and symptomatic adults. JAMA 2008;299:1027–35.
3. Goetz M, Wang TD. Molecular imaging in gastrointestinal endoscopy. Gastroenterology 2010;138:828–33.
4. Uedo N, Higashino K, Ishihara R, et al. Diagnosis of colonic adenomas by new autofluorescence imaging system: a pilot study. Dig Endosc 2007;19:S134–8.
5. Wang TD, Friedland S, Sahbaie P, et al. Functional imaging of colonic mucosa with a fibered confocal microscope for real time in vivo pathology. Clin Gastroenterol Hepatol 2007;5:1300–5.
6. Hsiung PL, Wang TD. *In vivo* biomarkers for targeting colorectal neoplasms. Cancer Biomark 2008;4:329–40.
7. Hsiung P, Hardy J, Friedland S, et al. Detection of colonic dysplasia in vivo using a targeted heptapeptide and confocal microendoscopy. Nat Med 2008;14:454–8.

Index

Note: Page numbers of article titles are in **boldface** type.

A

Adenoma(s)
  flat
    detection of, development of expertise in, procedure for, 453–454
    treatment of, 454–455
  polypoid, CRCs due to, 417
  serrated, **543–563**
    classification of, 544
    clinical implications of, 554–556
    endoscopic features of, 544–545
    histologic features of, 545–549
    hyperplastic, histologic features of, 545–546
    MAPK-ERK pathway alterations in, 550–554. See also *MAPK-ERK pathway alterations, in serrated adenomas.*
    mixed, histologic features of, 547–549
    molecular biologic changes in, 549–550
    morphologic features of, 544
    pathway of, 550
    sessile, histologic features of, 546–547
    traditional, histologic features of, 546
AFI. See *Autofluorescence imaging (AFI).*
Anticoagulant(s)
  cessation of, before ESD of NP-CRNs, 516
  management of, in EMR of NP-CRNs, 505–506
Antiplatelet agents
  cessation of, before ESD of NP-CRNs, 516
  management of, in EMR of NP-CRNs, 505–506
Apoptosis, regulation of, in serrated adenomas, alterations in, 552
Autofluorescence imaging (AFI), Olympus, in IEE for NP-CRNs, 476

B

Bacterial endocarditis, patients at high risk for, management of, before EMR of NP-CRNs, 506–507
Barium enema, in estimation of submucosal invasion in NP-CRNs, 488
Bowel preparation, in NP-CRNs detection, **439–442.** See also *Non-polypoid colorectal neoplasms (NP-CRNs), detection of, bowel preparation in.*
BRAF mutation, in serrated adenomas, 551

C

CAD. See *Computer-aided detection (CAD).*
Cancer(s)
  colorectal. See *Colorectal cancers (CRCs).*

Cancer(s) (*continued*)
    flat, prevalence of, 426
Chromoendoscopy, magnifying, in estimation of submucosal invasion in NP-CRNs, 491–494
Chromosome 17p, APC and LOH at chromosome 17p, 574–575
Colitis, ulcerative. See *Ulcerative colitis.*
Colon polyps, serrated, **543–563.** See also *Adenoma(s), serrated.*
Colonoscopy
    conventional, in estimation of submucosal invasion in NP-CRNs, 490
    in CRC prevention, 407–408
    in NP-CRN detection, 432
        patient preparation for, 442–443
    quality of. See also *Non-polypoid colorectal neoplasms, quality of colonoscopy and, relationship between.*
        indicators for, 508–509
        relationship to NP-CRNs, **407–415**
    surveillance, in NP-CRNs management in ulcerative colitis, 536–539
Colorectal cancers (CRCs)
    interval, 409–411
    intramucosal, treatment of, EMR in, 487
    macroscopic classification of, **461–469**
        basic principles of, 462–466
        clinical significance of, 466–467
        described, 461–462
        distinguishing depressed area of 0–IIc type lesion, 465–466
        endoscopic, 462–463
        flat lesion vs. 0–IIc type lesion, 463–465
    polypoid adenomas and, 417
    prevalence of, 449
    prevention of, colonoscopy in, 407–408
Colorectal lesions, diagnosis of, IEE in, 482–483
Computed tomographic colonography (CTC)
    NP-CRNs and, **565–572**
    of flat polyps
        technique for, 567–569
        with CAD, 569–570
    performance characteristics of, 566
Computeraided detection (CAD), CTC with, of flat polyps, 569–570
Conventional colonoscopy, in estimation of submucosal invasion in NP-CRNs, 490
CRCs. See *Colorectal cancers (CRCs).*
Crystal violet dye, in IEE for NP-CRNs, 474
CTC. See *Computed tomographic colonography (CTC).*

D

Depressed colonic neoplasms, targeted imaging of, **579–583**
    future challenges related to, 582–583
    instrumentation in, 580–581
    molecular probes in, 580
    results of, 581–582
DNA methylation, alterations related to, in serrated adenomas, 552–553
Dye-based IEE, of NP-CRNs, 474

in ulcerative colitis, 527–530

Dysplasia(s), in ulcerative colitis, histologic classification of, 534–536

Dysplasia-associated lesions or masses, in ulcerative colitis, vs. NP-CRNs, 532

E

EMR. See *Endoscopic mucosal resection (EMR)*.

Endocarditis, bacterial, patients at high risk for, management of, before EMR of NP-CRNs, 506–507

Endoscopic mucosal resection (EMR)
  for intramucosal CRC, 487
  of NP-CRNs, **503–514**
    anticoagulants in, management of, 505–506
    antiplatelets in, management of, 505–506
    clinical outcomes of, 512–513
    complications of, 513
    depth of invasion estimation in, 504–505
    described, 503
    detailed inject-and-cut procedure, 507–512
      "dynamic" submucosal injection, 507–508
      reassessment, 509–511
      snare, 508–509
      specimen retrieval and preparation, 511
      surveillance colonoscopy, 511–512
    in patients at high-risk for bacterial endocarditis, management of, 506–507
    indications for, 503–504
    vs. ESD, 520–522

Endoscopic submucosal dissection (ESD), of NP–CRNs, **515–524**
  at NCCH, Tokyo, 516–520
  care following, 522
  cessation of anticoagulants and antiplatelets before, 516
  clinical outcome of, 518
  complications of, 518–520
  depth of invasion estimation in, 516
  described, 515–516
  detailed procedures, 517–518
  indications for, 516
  submucosal injection solution in, 517
  vs. EMR, 520–522

Endoscopic ultrasonography, in estimation of submucosal invasion in NP-CRNs, 489–490

Endoscopist(s), learning curve for, NP-CRNs–detection related, 455–456

Endoscopy, IEE, for NP-CRNs, **471–485**. See also *Non-polypoid colorectal neoplasms (NP-CRNs), IEE in*.

Enema, barium, in estimation of submucosal invasion in NP-CRNs, 488

EPHB2 alterations, in serrated adenomas, 551–552

Equipment-based IEE, of NP-CRNs in ulcerative colitis, 530–531

ESD. See *Endoscopic submucosal dissection (ESD)*.

F

FICE. See *Fujinon intelligence color enhancement (FICE)*.

Flat nonneoplastic lesions, in ulcerative colitis, vs. NP-CRNs, 533–534

Flat polyps
    defined, 565–566
    detection of
        development of expertise in, procedure for, 453–454
        technique for, 567–569
    targeted imaging of, **579–583**
        future challenges related to, 582–583
        instrumentation in, 580–581
        molecular probes in, 580
        results of, 581–582
Fujinon intelligence color enhancement (FICE), in IEE for NP-CRNs, 474

G

Genetic(s), of NP-CRNs, **573–578.** See also *Non-polyploid colorectal neoplasms (NP-CRNs), genetic aspects of.*
Genome-wide transcriptional analysis, in NP-CRNs, 576

H

Hereditary nonpolyposis colorectal cancer (HNPCC) syndrome, IEE in, 481–482
HNPCC syndrome. See *Hereditary nonpolyposis colorectal cancer (HNPCC) syndrome.*
Hyperplastic polyposis, histologic features of, 549

I

IEE. See *Image-enhanced endoscopy (IEE).*
Image-enhanced endoscopy (IEE), for NP-CRNs, **471–485.** See also *Non-polyploid colorectal neoplasms (NP-CRNs), IEE in.*
    in ulcerative colitis, 527–531
        dye-based, 527–530
        equipment-based, 530–531
Indigo carmine dye, in IEE for NP-CRNs, 474

J

Japan polyp study, 434

K

K-*ras* mutations
    in serrated adenomas, 550–551
    RAS pathway and, 574

M

Magnifying chromoendoscopy, in estimation of submucosal invasion in NP-CRNs, 491–494
MAPK-ERK pathway alterations, in serrated adenomas, 550–554
    apoptosis regulation–related, 552
    BRAF mutation, 551
    DNA methylation–related, 552–553

EPHB2 alterations, 551–552
KRAS mutation, 550–551
MGMT alterations, 553
MSI and DNA mismatch repair abnormalities, 553
MGMT alterations, in serrated adenomas, 553
MSI and DNA mismatch repair abnormalities, in serrated adenomas, 553
Mutation(s)
    in serrated adenomas, 551
    K-*ras, RAS* pathway and, 574

N

Narrow band imaging (NBI), Olympus, in IEE for NP-CRNs, 475
National Cancer Center Hospital (NCCH), Tokyo, data from, in estimation of submucosal
    invasion in NP-CRNs, 490–491
NBI. See *Narrow band imaging (NBI).*
NCCH. See *National Cancer Center Hospital (NCCH).*
Neoplasm(s), colorectal, macroscopic classification of, importance of, **461–469.** See also
    Colorectal cancers (CRCs), macroscopic classification of.
Nonlifting sign, in estimation of submucosal invasion in NP-CRNs, 490
Non-polypoid colorectal neoplasms (NP-CRNs)
    among ulcerative colitis–related neoplasias, prevalence of, 526–527
    analysis of, colonoscopic, 432
    biological significance of, 419–426
    classification of, development of expertise in, **449–460**
    CTC and, **565–572**
    depressed-type, importance of, 432–433
    detection of
        bowel preparation in, **439–442**
            assessment of, 439–440
            customization of preparation, 442
            diet on day before procedure in, 442
            improvement of, 440–442
            patient education in, 442
            solutions for, 439
            split-dose regimen in, 440–441
            timing of colonoscopy after inadequate preparation, 442
        colonoscopy in
            patient preparation for, 442–443
            procedure, 443–445
            quality of, **407–415**
                described, 411–413
        development of expertise in, **449–460**
            importance of, 451–453
        endoscopic recognition in, 437–438
        learning pyramid related to, 450–451
    EMR of, **503–514.** See also *Endoscopic mucosal resection (EMR), of NP-CRNs.*
    ESD of, **515–524.** See also *Endoscopic submucosal dissection (ESD), of NP-CRNs.*
    evaluation of, radiographic, 431–432
    genetic aspects of, **573–578**
        animal models, development of, 576

Non-polypoid (*continued*)
    APC and LOH at chromosome 17p, 574–575
    described, 573
    future directions in, 576
    genome-wide transcriptional analysis, 576
    K-*ras* mutations, 574
    microsatellite instability and methylation, 575–576
    molecular correlates of tumor behavior, 575
  IEE in, **471–485**
    average-risk screening, 480–481
    colorectal lesions, 482–483
    described, 471–473
    high-risk screening, 481–482
    in colon and rectum, in authors' practice, 477–479
      supporting literature for, 479–483
    in HNPCC syndrome, 481–482
    in ulcerative colitis, 481
    techniques, 474–477
      dye-based, 474
      equipment-based, 474–477
      FICE, 474
      Olympus AFI, 476
      Olympus NBI, 475
      Pentax iScan, 476–477
  in ulcerative colitis, **525–542.** See also *Ulcerative colitis, NP-CRNs in.*
  Japan polyp study, 434
  natural history of, **431–435**
  prevalence of, worldwide, **417–429**
    Asia, 418
    flat cancers, 426
    variation in, reasons for, 418–419
    western countries, 418
  submucosal invasion in, estimation of, **487–496**
    barium enema in, 488
    conventional colonoscopy in, 490
    data from NCCH, Tokyo in, 490–491
    endoscopic ultrasonography in, 489–490
    importance of, 488
    magnifying chromoendoscopy in, 491–494
    nonlifting sign in, 490
  unanswered questions about, 457
NP-CRNs. See *Non-polypoid colorectal neoplasms (NP-CRNs).*

O

Olympus AFI, in IEE for NP-CRNs, 476
Olympus NBI, in IEE for NP-CRNs, 475

P

Pentax iScan, in IEE for NP-CRNs, 476–477
Pit patterns, in NP-CRNs in ulcerative colitis, 531–532

Polyp(s)
    colon, serrated, **543–563.** See also *Adenoma(s), serrated.*
    flat. See *Flat polyps.*
Polypoid adenomas, CRCs due to, 417
Polyposis, hyperplastic, histologic features of, 549

R

RAS pathway, K-*ras* mutations and, 574

S

Serrated neoplasia pathway, 550, 554
Submucosal injection technique, **497–502**
    described, 497
    dynamic, 499–501
    static, 497–498

U

Ulcerative colitis
    dysplasia in, histologic classification of, 534–536
    neoplastic and dysplastic lesions in, IEE of, 481
    NP-CRNs in, **525–542**
        described, 525
        detection of, 527
        diagnosis of, 527
        equipment-based, 530–531
        IEE of, 527–531
        management of, 534–539
            surveillance colonoscopy in, 536–539
        pit patterns in, 531–532
        prevalence of, 525–526
        vs. dysplasia-associated lesions or masses, 532
        vs. flat nonneoplastic lesions, 533–534
Ulcerative colitis–related neoplasias, NP-CRNs among, prevalence of, 526–527
Ultrasonography, endoscopic, in estimation of submucosal invasion in NP-CRNs, 489–490

Z

0-IIc lesions
    depressed area of, distinguishing of, 465–466
    flat lesions vs., 463–465
    pathologic features of, 466–467
    prevalence of, 466–467

Printed and bound by CPI Group (UK) Ltd, Croydon, CR0 4YY

03/10/2024

01040454-0016